Barbara Jones

The Castor Oil Bible

Your All-in-One Guide to Natural Healing, Beauty & Detox with 300 Easy Recipes for Visible Results in 7 Days.

ARIES PUBLISHING LLC

ISBN: 979-8-89843-158-7

Table of Contents

Chapter 1: Introduction to Castor Oil

Chapter 2: Skin Rejuvenation with Castor Oil

Chapter 3: Transforming Hair with Castor Oil

Chapter 4: Enhancing Brows and Lashes

Chapter 5: Complete Body Care

Chapter 6: Pain and Inflammation Relief

Chapter 7: Women's Health Remedies

Chapter 8: Total Body Detox and Gut Health

Chapter 9: Crafting with Castor Oil

Chapter 10: Incorporating Castor Oil into Daily Routine

Chapter 11: Holistic Healing: Beyond Castor Oil

Chapter 12: Real-Life Transformations

Chapter 1: Introduction to Castor Oil

Castor oil, derived from the seeds of the Ricinus communis plant, boasts a storied history that dates back thousands of years, weaving its way through various cultures and civilizations. This ancient oil is not merely a modern trend; rather, it has been revered for its myriad of uses, both medicinal and cosmetic, across different eras. Exploring its origins provides a fascinating glimpse into how this simple oil has become a cornerstone of natural healing and beauty practices.

The use of castor oil can be traced back to ancient Egypt, where it was prized not only for its healing properties but also for its role in beauty rituals. The Egyptians utilized castor oil as a natural moisturizer and as a base for cosmetics. Evidence suggests that Cleopatra herself may have employed it in her beauty regimen, enhancing her allure with the help of this golden oil. Beyond beauty, castor oil was also used in the embalming process, highlighting its significance in ritualistic practices surrounding death and the afterlife.

As we venture beyond Egypt, the oil found its way into the medicinal practices of ancient India, where it was known as "Eranda." Ayurveda, the traditional Indian system of medicine, harnesses the therapeutic properties of castor oil for various ailments. Ancient texts describe its usage as a purgative, promoting digestive health and detoxification. The oil was also applied topically to soothe skin conditions and promote hair growth, showcasing its versatility as both a health and beauty remedy.

In the Greco-Roman world, castor oil continued to be held in high esteem. The Greek physician Hippocrates, often referred to as the "Father of Medicine," wrote about the oil's benefits, particularly its laxative properties. The Romans utilized castor oil in their baths, appreciating its ability to soften skin and maintain a youthful appearance. This practice laid the groundwork for contemporary uses of castor oil in skincare, as its emollient qualities were recognized long before the advent of modern cosmetics.

The spread of castor oil across continents continued through trade routes, reaching Africa, Asia, and eventually the Americas. In Africa, castor oil became integral to traditional healing practices, utilized for its anti-inflammatory properties and as a treatment for wounds and infections. Indigenous tribes embraced the oil, recognizing its efficacy in promoting overall health and wellness. This deep-rooted appreciation for castor oil as a natural remedy endures in many African cultures today.

During the 18th and 19th centuries, castor oil gained popularity in Western medicine. It was commonly prescribed as a laxative and a remedy for various ailments, from digestive issues to skin irritations. Its popularity surged during times of war, as castor oil was recognized for its ability to alleviate discomfort and promote healing in wounded soldiers. The oil's reputation as a beneficial remedy was solidified, and it became a staple in many households.

However, the 20th century brought about a significant shift in the perception of castor oil. As synthetic alternatives flooded the market, the oil's traditional uses began to wane. Chemical-laden products dominated the beauty and healthcare industries, overshadowing the natural remedies that had been revered for centuries. Despite this, castor oil never entirely fell out of favor; it remained a beloved staple in the homes of those who valued its natural properties.

The resurgence of interest in natural and holistic health practices in recent years has led to a renaissance of castor oil. As people become increasingly aware of the potential dangers of synthetic chemicals and pharmaceuticals, they are turning back to nature for solutions. This renewed recognition of castor oil's versatility has sparked a modern revival, with individuals seeking out its benefits for skincare, haircare, and overall wellness.

The scientific community has also begun to catch up with the wisdom of ancient traditions. Research studies have delved into the composition of castor oil, revealing its rich content of ricinoleic acid—a fatty acid known for its anti-inflammatory, analgesic, and antimicrobial properties. This scientific validation has reinforced the oil's reputation as a natural remedy, further enticing a new generation of users to explore its potential.

Today, castor oil is celebrated not only for its historical significance but also for its practicality in addressing contemporary health and beauty concerns. Whether used to combat acne, promote hair growth, or alleviate joint pain, this oil has proven itself time and again as a reliable ally to those seeking natural solutions.

As we embark on a journey through "The Castor Oil Bible," it is essential to appreciate the rich tapestry of history that surrounds this remarkable oil. The stories of ancient civilizations, the wisdom of herbal medicine, and the scientific discoveries of modern times converge to highlight the enduring significance of castor oil. By embracing this age-old remedy, we honor the generations that have come before us, while also empowering ourselves to take charge of our health and beauty in a natural, sustainable way.

Incorporating castor oil into your daily routine is not just about using a beneficial product; it’s about connecting with a legacy that spans across cultures and centuries. It’s about tapping into the earth's resources and allowing nature to guide us toward holistic well-being. As we continue our exploration in the chapters that follow, remember that with each drop of castor oil, you are participating in a time-honored tradition of healing and self-care that has stood the test of time. Embrace this golden oil, and unlock the potential that awaits you on your journey to a healthier, more radiant you.

The allure of castor oil lies not only in its rich history but also in its remarkable effectiveness, supported by a growing body of scientific research. As we delve into the mechanisms of how castor oil works, it becomes clear why this simple, natural substance has stood the test of time and continues to be a favored remedy in the modern age.

At the heart of castor oil's efficacy is its primary component, ricinoleic acid. This unique fatty acid comprises about 90% of castor oil's composition, setting it apart from other vegetable oils. Ricinoleic acid possesses anti-inflammatory, analgesic, and antimicrobial properties, which contribute significantly to its therapeutic effects. Scientific studies have demonstrated that this compound can inhibit the activity of certain inflammatory mediators, making it an effective natural remedy for alleviating pain and swelling. When applied topically, ricinoleic acid penetrates the skin barrier, allowing it to reach deeper layers where inflammation often resides, thereby providing relief for conditions like arthritis and muscle soreness.

The moisturizing capabilities of castor oil are another aspect rooted in science. Its high viscosity and unique structure allow it to create a protective barrier on the skin, preventing moisture loss. This occlusive property is beneficial for maintaining hydration, especially in dry skin conditions. Furthermore, castor oil's emollient characteristics help to soften and soothe the skin, making it an excellent choice for those dealing with rough patches, dryness, and irritation. Research has shown that fatty acids, such as those found in castor oil, are integral to maintaining the skin's lipid barrier, which is essential for overall skin health.

In addition to its effects on the skin, castor oil has demonstrated positive outcomes in hair care. The application of ricinoleic acid not only nourishes the scalp but also stimulates the hair follicles, promoting healthier hair growth. Studies have indicated that the fatty acid supports blood circulation, which is vital for delivering nutrients to hair follicles. Improved blood flow can lead to stronger, thicker hair and may help combat hair loss. The oil's antifungal properties also make it effective against scalp conditions like dandruff, ensuring a healthy environment for hair to thrive.

The versatility of castor oil extends to its benefits for digestive health as well. When ingested, ricinoleic acid acts as a potent laxative, promoting bowel movement by stimulating intestinal contractions. This natural laxative effect has been substantiated by numerous studies and has made castor oil a popular choice for those seeking relief from constipation without the use of synthetic medications. The oil also supports liver function, helping to detoxify the body and improve overall gut health. By enhancing the digestive process and promoting regularity, castor oil serves as a gentle yet effective approach to maintaining a healthy digestive system.

Moreover, the antimicrobial properties of castor oil offer protection against various pathogens. Research has shown that castor oil can inhibit the growth of certain bacteria and fungi, making it a valuable ally in preventing infections and promoting skin health. Its ability to combat microbes is particularly beneficial in the treatment of minor cuts, abrasions, and skin irritations, as it can help to prevent infection while facilitating healing.

The science behind castor oil is further supported by its historical application in traditional medicine across various cultures. Ancient Egyptians used it for skin ailments and as a laxative, while traditional Ayurvedic practices in India have lauded its benefits for hair and skin care for centuries. This long-standing usage provides a strong foundation for the modern scientific validation of castor oil's effectiveness.

As we navigate the world of self-care and natural remedies, the importance of understanding the science behind them cannot be overstated. Castor oil stands out as a prime example of how nature can provide effective solutions for common health and beauty concerns. Its multifaceted benefits, backed by scientific evidence, make it a go-to ingredient for those seeking to enhance their well-being naturally.

Incorporating castor oil into your daily routine not only offers a wealth of benefits but also allows you to harness the power of nature to foster self-healing. Whether you're looking to rejuvenate your skin, promote hair growth, alleviate discomfort, or improve digestive health, castor oil provides a holistic approach that resonates with the principles of natural wellness. The synergy of its components, particularly ricinoleic acid, showcases the profound impact that a single ingredient can have on multiple facets of health.

Ultimately, the scientific backing of castor oil reinforces its place in the realm of natural remedies. It empowers individuals to make informed choices about their health and beauty regimens while embracing the simplicity of nature's offerings. As we move forward in this exploration of castor oil's capabilities, let us celebrate the intersection of ancient wisdom and modern science, and recognize the potential that lies within this golden oil, ready to transform our lives for the better.

When it comes to natural remedies, few substances generate as much intrigue and skepticism as castor oil. Despite its long history of use and the growing body of scientific support for its benefits, misconceptions abound. Understanding these myths is essential, as it allows individuals to make informed decisions about incorporating castor oil into their health and beauty routines. Here, we will unravel some of the most prevalent myths surrounding castor oil, clarifying its properties, uses, and benefits.

One of the most common misconceptions is that castor oil is only suitable for hair and skin treatments. This belief stems from its popularity in beauty circles, where it is often touted as a miracle worker for hair growth and skin hydration. While it's true that castor oil excels in these areas due to its rich fatty acid content and moisturizing properties, its benefits extend far beyond aesthetics. Castor oil has been used for centuries in traditional medicine to alleviate digestive issues, relieve joint pain, and even support women's health. The oil's unique composition makes it a versatile remedy that can be utilized in various ways, addressing not just external beauty concerns but internal health as well.

Another myth is that castor oil is too heavy and greasy for regular use, especially on the skin. This perception likely arises from its thick, viscous texture. However, many users find that once applied, castor oil absorbs surprisingly well, leaving the skin feeling soft and nourished rather than greasy. The key is to use it in moderation and to combine it with lighter oils or other ingredients if desired. For instance, mixing castor oil with jojoba or almond oil can create a lighter blend that retains all the benefits without the heaviness. Furthermore, castor oil can be an excellent carrier oil for essential oils, enhancing their absorption and potency when applied topically.

Some individuals assume that castor oil is only suitable for specific skin types, particularly dry or damaged skin. This belief can deter those with oily or sensitive skin from trying it. Contrary to this myth, castor oil can actually be beneficial for all skin types. Its antibacterial and anti-inflammatory properties make it a great choice for oily or acne-prone skin, as it can help reduce breakouts and soothe irritation. Additionally, those with sensitive skin may find that castor oil acts as a gentle moisturizer without causing adverse reactions, provided they perform a patch test before widespread application.

There's also a misconception that castor oil is a modern trend with no historical basis. In reality, castor oil has been used for thousands of years, tracing back to ancient Egypt, where it was revered for its medicinal and cosmetic properties. Egyptian queens reportedly used it as part of their beauty rituals, while it was also prescribed for various ailments. In traditional Indian medicine, castor oil is known as "Eranda oil" and is utilized for its health benefits, including acting as a laxative and promoting digestive health. This rich history underscores the reliability of castor oil as a time-tested remedy rather than a fleeting fad.

Another myth revolves around the idea that castor oil is unsafe for internal use. While it's true that consuming castor oil in excessive amounts can lead to unpleasant side effects, such as cramping or diarrhea, when used correctly, it is generally considered safe. Many people use it as a natural laxative to relieve constipation, but it's crucial to follow recommended dosages and consult a healthcare professional if you have any underlying health conditions. Understanding the appropriate uses and dosages is key to enjoying castor oil's benefits without adverse effects.

Some believe that castor oil's effectiveness is purely anecdotal, lacking scientific support. However, recent studies have begun to validate many of the claims made about castor oil. Research has demonstrated its anti-inflammatory and analgesic properties, making it effective for reducing pain and inflammation. Other studies have shown its potential benefits in promoting hair growth, soothing dry skin, and even supporting immune function. While more research is needed to explore the full extent of its benefits, the existing body of evidence supports the idea that castor oil is more than just an old wives' tale.

Additionally, there's a misconception that all castor oil products are created equal. Not all castor oil is of the same quality, and the extraction method can significantly impact its efficacy. Cold-pressed, organic castor oil retains more nutrients and beneficial properties compared to refined versions, which may undergo chemical processing that strips away some of its natural benefits. When selecting castor oil for personal use, it's essential to choose high-quality, pure, and preferably organic products to ensure the best results.

Lastly, some individuals believe that castor oil can lead to allergic reactions or skin irritation. While it is true that some people may be sensitive to castor oil, such occurrences are relatively rare. The best way to determine if you will have a reaction is to conduct a patch test on a small area of skin before applying it more widely. This precaution helps identify any sensitivities, allowing you to enjoy the benefits of castor oil safely.

In conclusion, while castor oil is surrounded by myths and misconceptions, a deeper understanding of its history, properties, and uses reveals its true potential as a natural remedy. By dispelling these myths, you can confidently explore the myriad ways castor oil can enhance your health and beauty routine, empowering you to embrace a more holistic approach to wellness. Whether you're looking to rejuvenate your skin, boost hair growth, or promote internal health, castor oil might just be the golden solution you've been seeking.

Chapter 2: Skin Rejuvenation with Castor Oil

Acne and blemishes can be a source of frustration and insecurity for many, often leading to an endless cycle of trying various products that promise clear skin but fail to deliver. The good news is that nature offers effective solutions, and castor oil is one of the most versatile and powerful ingredients you can incorporate into your skincare routine. Its unique properties not only help combat acne but also promote overall skin health, making it a must-have in your natural remedy arsenal.

Castor oil is rich in ricinoleic acid, a fatty acid with potent anti-inflammatory and antimicrobial properties. This makes it particularly effective in treating acne, as it helps to reduce the swelling and redness associated with breakouts while fighting off the bacteria that can worsen skin conditions. Additionally, castor oil is a humectant, meaning it draws moisture into the skin, providing hydration without clogging pores. This unique combination of benefits makes castor oil an ideal choice for those looking to achieve a clearer, healthier complexion.

To harness the power of castor oil for acne and blemishes, consider the following DIY treatments that are simple to prepare and incorporate into your skincare routine.

One of the most straightforward methods is to use castor oil as a spot treatment. Simply apply a small amount of pure castor oil directly to the affected areas using a cotton swab. This concentrated application allows the oil to penetrate the skin and deliver its healing properties directly where they are needed most. For best results, apply this treatment before bedtime and allow it to work overnight. You'll wake up to calmer, less inflamed skin.

For those with more widespread acne or blemishes, a castor oil facial mask can be an excellent option. Combine one tablespoon of castor oil with one tablespoon of honey, a natural antibacterial and humectant that complements the healing properties of castor oil. Mix the two ingredients until well blended, and apply an even layer to your face, avoiding the eye area. Leave the mask on for 20 to 30 minutes to allow the nutrients to penetrate the skin, then rinse off with warm water. This mask not only helps to reduce acne but also leaves your skin feeling soft and hydrated.

Another effective treatment involves the addition of essential oils to castor oil. Tea tree oil, for instance, is renowned for its acne-fighting properties due to its strong antibacterial and anti-inflammatory effects. To create a potent acne-fighting blend, mix one tablespoon of castor oil with five drops of tea tree oil. Apply this combination to your blemishes, and let it sit for at least 30 minutes before rinsing. This powerful duo can help reduce the appearance of acne while preventing future breakouts.

For those who prefer a more comprehensive approach, consider creating a castor oil cleansing routine. Begin by mixing two tablespoons of castor oil with one tablespoon of a carrier oil, such as jojoba or sweet almond oil. This blend will not only help to cleanse your skin of impurities and makeup but also provide nourishment and hydration. Massage the mixture onto dry skin, focusing on areas prone to breakouts, and then use a warm, damp washcloth to gently wipe away the oil. This method effectively removes dirt and excess sebum without stripping the skin of its natural oils, making it a great option for those with acne-prone skin.

In addition to topical treatments, it's essential to consider the role of diet and overall wellness in managing acne. Incorporating castor oil into your diet can provide internal benefits that promote healthier skin from within. Try taking one teaspoon of cold-pressed castor oil daily, either on its own or mixed with a smoothie or juice. This can help to improve digestion, reduce inflammation, and support overall skin health.

When using castor oil for acne and blemishes, it's important to remember that consistency is key. Results may not be immediate; however, with regular use, many people find that their skin begins to clear and improve over time. Patience and persistence are essential, as is paying attention to how your skin responds to the treatments. Everyone's skin is unique, so it may take some experimentation to find the right routine for your individual needs.

Before diving into any new skincare regimen, it's advisable to perform a patch test, especially if you have sensitive skin. Apply a small amount of castor oil to a discreet area and observe for any adverse reactions over 24 hours. If you experience redness, itching, or irritation, it may be best to adjust your approach and consult with a dermatologist if necessary.

While castor oil is a remarkable natural remedy for acne and blemishes, it is essential to complement its use with a healthy lifestyle. Staying hydrated, eating a balanced diet rich in fruits and vegetables, and managing stress levels can significantly impact your skin's health. Regular exercise also promotes circulation, which can help deliver oxygen and nutrients to your skin, further enhancing its appearance.

As you embark on your journey to clearer skin with castor oil, remember that natural remedies often take time to show results. Embrace the process and enjoy the ritual of self-care that accompanies using these treatments. With dedication and the right approach, you can achieve the radiant, blemish-free skin you desire—one drop of castor oil at a time.

As we age, our skin undergoes a myriad of changes, often manifesting as fine lines, wrinkles, and a loss of elasticity. While many turn to expensive creams and invasive procedures in search of a more youthful appearance, the solution may lie in a simple, natural remedy: castor oil. This golden oil, derived from the seeds of the castor bean plant, has been celebrated for centuries for its remarkable skin benefits. In this section, we will explore how castor oil can help reduce wrinkles and provide deep hydration, allowing you to embrace a more radiant complexion.

The primary component of castor oil is ricinoleic acid, a monounsaturated fatty acid that possesses anti-inflammatory and moisturizing properties. This unique composition allows castor oil to penetrate deeply into the skin, delivering essential nutrients while promoting hydration at the cellular level. Unlike many commercial moisturizers that may contain harsh chemicals, castor oil is gentle on the skin, making it suitable for even the most sensitive types. Its ability to mimic the skin's natural sebum helps restore the moisture barrier, preventing dryness and the formation of fine lines.

One of the most effective ways to harness the anti-aging benefits of castor oil is through regular application as part of your evening skincare routine. Begin by cleansing your face thoroughly to remove makeup, dirt, and impurities. Once your skin is clean, take a few drops of castor oil and warm it between your palms. This will help activate its soothing properties. Gently massage the oil into your skin using upward circular motions, focusing on areas prone to wrinkles, such as the forehead, around the eyes, and the corners of the mouth.

For enhanced effectiveness, consider combining castor oil with other natural ingredients known for their anti-aging properties. For instance, mixing castor oil with a few drops of essential oils like frankincense or lavender can further boost its rejuvenating effects. Frankincense is renowned for its ability to reduce the appearance of fine lines and improve skin tone, while lavender offers soothing properties that can help reduce stress and promote restful sleep. Simply blend a few drops of your chosen essential oil with castor oil before application, and enjoy the aromatic benefits as you pamper your skin.

Another powerful combination is castor oil and vitamin E oil. Vitamin E is a potent antioxidant that helps protect the skin from damage caused by free radicals, which can accelerate the aging process. Mix equal parts of castor oil and vitamin E oil, and apply it nightly as a serum. The synergy between these two oils will not only hydrate your skin but also nourish it, promoting a plump and youthful appearance.

In addition to its hydrating properties, castor oil can also assist in reducing the appearance of existing wrinkles. Its emollient nature helps to fill in fine lines, making them less noticeable. For best results, consider using castor oil as an overnight treatment. Apply a thin layer to the affected areas before bed and allow it to work its magic while you sleep. You may wake up to noticeably softer, smoother skin, with fine lines appearing diminished.

Moreover, castor oil's anti-inflammatory properties can help soothe irritated skin, making it a fantastic option for those dealing with redness or inflammation associated with aging. By incorporating castor oil into your skincare routine, you're not only addressing wrinkles but also promoting overall skin health. The oil's natural composition can help balance oil production, making it beneficial for both dry and oily skin types.

For those who enjoy DIY skincare, consider creating a castor oil-based facial mask. Combine castor oil with natural ingredients such as honey and yogurt for a nourishing treatment that deeply hydrates and revitalizes the skin. Honey is a natural humectant, drawing moisture to the skin, while yogurt contains lactic acid, which gently exfoliates and brightens. Apply this mask once or twice a week for a rejuvenating boost that will leave your skin feeling refreshed and youthful.

It's essential to remember that consistency is key when it comes to seeing results. While you may notice immediate hydration and softness after the first application, the true benefits of castor oil will accumulate over time. Regular use will help improve skin texture, elasticity, and overall appearance. To track your progress, consider taking before and after photos, allowing you to visually appreciate the transformation that occurs with dedicated care.

As you embark on your journey to youthful skin with castor oil, it's also important to complement your external treatments with healthy lifestyle choices. Hydration, a balanced diet, and sun protection are crucial for maintaining skin health. Drinking plenty of water helps flush out toxins and keeps the skin plump, while a diet rich in antioxidants—from fruits, vegetables, and healthy fats—supports your skin from within. Additionally, always apply sunscreen during the day to shield your skin from harmful UV rays that contribute to premature aging.

Incorporating castor oil into your skincare routine is not merely about addressing wrinkles; it's about embracing a holistic approach to skin health. By choosing a natural, nourishing oil over chemical-laden products, you're actively participating in your skin's rejuvenation process. The simplicity and effectiveness of castor oil make it an invaluable addition to your beauty regimen.

As you begin to witness the transformation in your skin, you may find that castor oil becomes not just a remedy but a beloved staple in your self-care routine. Embrace the power of this ancient oil, and let it guide you toward achieving the glowing, youthful complexion you desire. With patience and persistence, castor oil can help you reclaim your skin's vitality and radiance, allowing you to face the world with confidence and grace.

The journey toward radiant skin often feels like navigating a maze filled with countless products, each promising miraculous results. Yet, amidst the confusion, one natural remedy emerges as a proven ally: castor oil. This ancient oil, derived from the seeds of the Ricinus communis plant, has been revered for its therapeutic properties for centuries. It’s time to shine a light on the various skin issues that castor oil can effectively address, helping you reclaim your confidence and embrace your natural beauty.

One of the most common concerns people face is acne. The relentless battle against breakouts can take a toll on self-esteem, and while many over-the-counter treatments are available, they can be harsh and drying. Castor oil offers a gentle yet potent alternative. Its rich composition includes ricinoleic acid, which possesses antibacterial properties that can help combat the bacteria responsible for acne. By applying a small amount of castor oil directly to affected areas, you can reduce inflammation and promote healing. For a more comprehensive approach, consider blending castor oil with tea tree oil, a well-known natural antiseptic. This combination can enhance the oil’s acne-fighting capabilities while soothing the skin.

Beyond acne, many struggle with uneven skin tone and hyperpigmentation. The natural emollient properties of castor oil make it an excellent choice for fading dark spots and promoting a more uniform complexion. The oil penetrates deeply into the skin, providing moisture and nourishment that encourage cell turnover. Incorporating castor oil into your nighttime skincare routine can work wonders. Simply dab a few drops onto dark spots before bed and allow the oil to work its magic overnight. Over time, you may notice a significant reduction in the appearance of blemishes, revealing a brighter, more radiant complexion.

For those grappling with dryness and rough patches, castor oil acts as a deeply hydrating agent. It forms a protective barrier on the skin, locking in moisture and preventing water loss. This is particularly beneficial during the colder months when skin tends to become parched. A simple castor oil body treatment can be incredibly effective: combine castor oil with a carrier oil like coconut or almond oil and massage it onto your skin after a shower. This not only replenishes moisture but also leaves your skin feeling silky smooth and rejuvenated.

Another skin issue many face is the appearance of fine lines and wrinkles associated with aging. The anti-inflammatory properties of castor oil can help reduce the visibility of these signs by promoting collagen production and improving skin elasticity. Regular application of castor oil around the eyes can help diminish crow's feet and puffiness. To create a nourishing eye treatment, mix castor oil with a few drops of rosehip oil, known for its rejuvenating properties. Gently pat the mixture around the delicate eye area each night, allowing the oils to penetrate and work their restorative magic while you sleep.

Sun exposure can wreak havoc on the skin, leading to sunburns and premature aging. If you've spent too long in the sun and are dealing with red, irritated skin, castor oil can provide relief. Its anti-inflammatory properties help soothe the burn, while its moisturizing effect can alleviate the dryness that often follows. To create a soothing sunburn remedy, mix castor oil with aloe vera gel, which further cools and hydrates the skin. Apply this blend to the affected areas to promote healing and prevent peeling.

In addition to these more common issues, some individuals may experience skin conditions such as eczema or psoriasis, which can cause chronic discomfort and embarrassment. While these conditions can be complex and often require medical intervention, castor oil can serve as a supportive treatment. Its anti-inflammatory and moisturizing properties can provide temporary relief from the itching and irritation associated with these conditions. Apply castor oil directly to the affected areas or mix it with a soothing essential oil like lavender for added calming effects.

Dry, cracked heels can also be a significant issue, particularly for those who spend long hours on their feet. Castor oil can help restore softness and prevent further cracking. Before bed, massage a generous amount of castor oil into your feet, paying special attention to the heels. For maximum effectiveness, wear cotton socks afterward to allow the oil to penetrate overnight. By morning, you'll notice an improvement in texture, and with consistent application, you can maintain soft, supple feet.

Another often-overlooked benefit of castor oil is its role in reducing the appearance of scars. Whether from acne, injuries, or surgical procedures, scars can be a source of self-consciousness. The regenerative properties of castor oil can help improve the texture and appearance of scars over time. To create a targeted scar treatment, combine castor oil with vitamin E oil, known for its skin-healing properties. Apply this mixture to the scarred area and massage gently, encouraging absorption and stimulating circulation.

Lastly, let's not forget the power of castor oil in the battle against dry and chapped lips. The same hydrating qualities that benefit your skin can also work wonders for your lips. A simple lip balm can be made by combining castor oil with beeswax and a few drops of your favorite essential oil for flavor. This luxurious balm will keep your lips moisturized and protected, making them soft and kissable.

Incorporating castor oil into your skincare routine can be a transformative experience. With its versatility and effectiveness, it addresses a myriad of skin concerns, providing natural solutions that empower you to achieve healthier, more vibrant skin. As you explore the wonders of this golden oil, remember that consistency is key. With patience and dedication, you'll discover the profound impact castor oil can have on your skin, helping you embrace your beauty with confidence.

Chapter 3: Transforming Hair with Castor Oil

Unruly hair, thinning locks, and excessive shedding can be sources of distress for many individuals. Whether you're dealing with seasonal shedding, stress-related hair loss, or simply the effects of aging, the quest for fuller, healthier hair can feel overwhelming. Fortunately, nature has equipped us with powerful tools, and castor oil stands out as one of the most effective and versatile options available for stimulating hair growth naturally.

Castor oil is derived from the seeds of the Ricinus communis plant and has been used for centuries for its therapeutic properties. Its rich composition of fatty acids, particularly ricinoleic acid, plays a crucial role in promoting hair growth. This unique fatty acid enhances blood circulation to the scalp, which is essential for delivering oxygen and nutrients to hair follicles. Improved circulation stimulates hair growth and can lead to thicker, healthier strands over time.

One of the most compelling aspects of castor oil is its ability to moisturize the scalp and hair. Dandruff and dry scalp can hinder hair growth, leading to breakage and stunted growth. The deep moisturizing properties of castor oil penetrate the hair shaft, providing essential hydration that keeps both the scalp and hair nourished. Unlike many commercial hair products that contain harsh chemicals, castor oil offers a natural alternative that is gentle yet effective.

To harness the hair growth benefits of castor oil, you can create a simple yet powerful hair treatment at home. Begin with pure castor oil; organic, cold-pressed varieties are preferred to ensure you receive the maximum benefits. While castor oil can be thick and sticky, you can mix it with lighter oils such as coconut oil or jojoba oil to create a more manageable blend. These oils not only enhance the application process but also add additional nutrients that promote hair health.

For a rejuvenating scalp treatment, warm the oil blend slightly—this enhances absorption and promotes relaxation. Section your hair and apply the oil directly to your scalp using your fingertips. Gently massage the oil into your scalp in circular motions for about five to ten minutes. This massage not only stimulates circulation but also promotes relaxation, which can alleviate stress—a known factor in hair loss.

Once your scalp is treated, you can distribute the remaining oil through the lengths of your hair. This is especially beneficial for the ends, which are often the most damaged. After applying the oil, consider wrapping your hair in a warm towel or using a shower cap to create a warm environment that enhances absorption. Leave the treatment on for at least 30 minutes, but if time permits, overnight is even better. This allows your hair to soak up the nutrients fully.

After the treatment, wash your hair with a gentle, sulfate-free shampoo to remove excess oil. You may need to shampoo twice to ensure all the oil is removed, especially if you used a heavier blend. Follow with a conditioner to lock in moisture and improve manageability.

Incorporating castor oil into your hair care routine doesn't have to be a weekly endeavor—consider making it a part of your regimen. Regular treatments—once a week or every other week—can lead to noticeable improvements in hair thickness and growth.

Over time, you may find your hair feels more robust, looks shinier, and is less prone to breakage.

In addition to topical applications, consider consuming castor oil internally for additional benefits. While this should be approached with caution and ideally under the guidance of a healthcare professional, some individuals incorporate small amounts of castor oil into their diets for its laxative effects and potential detoxifying properties. This internal approach may support overall wellness, which can indirectly benefit hair health.

Another aspect of stimulating hair growth is understanding the importance of a balanced diet. Hair is primarily made up of protein, so ensuring you consume adequate amounts of protein-rich foods—like eggs, fish, nuts, and legumes—will provide the building blocks for strong hair. Additionally, vitamins and minerals play a crucial role in hair health. Biotin, zinc, iron, and vitamins A, C, D, and E are particularly important. A diet rich in fruits, vegetables, whole grains, and healthy fats will support not only your hair but your overall well-being.

Hydration is equally vital; drinking enough water daily ensures that your body is functioning optimally and can support hair growth. When your body is well-hydrated, your scalp remains moisturized, which promotes a healthier environment for hair to thrive.

Lastly, consider potential stressors that may be affecting your hair health. Chronic stress can lead to hair loss or thinning. Engage in stress-reducing activities that resonate with you, whether it's yoga, meditation, or simply taking time for self-care. Balancing your physical and mental well-being can significantly impact your hair's vitality.

In summary, stimulating hair growth naturally with castor oil is not just about the oil itself; it involves a holistic approach to hair care that includes nourishing your scalp, maintaining a balanced diet, staying hydrated, and managing stress. Through consistent application of castor oil, combined with healthy lifestyle choices, you can transform your hair from fragile and thinning to thick and vibrant. Embrace the power of castor oil as a key player in your journey to achieving the luscious locks you desire, and watch as your hair flourishes in response.

The health of your hair is intricately linked to the condition of your scalp. A well-nourished scalp not only promotes hair growth but also creates the ideal environment for strong, vibrant hair. One of the most prevalent issues affecting the scalp is dandruff, a condition that can be both embarrassing and frustrating. Luckily, castor oil is here to provide effective relief while nourishing your scalp and rejuvenating your hair.

Castor oil, derived from the seeds of the Ricinus communis plant, is rich in ricinoleic acid, a unique fatty acid that possesses powerful anti-inflammatory and antifungal properties. These qualities make it an excellent choice for addressing dandruff, which is often caused by an overgrowth of yeast on the scalp. When you apply castor oil to your scalp, you can target the root causes of dandruff, restoring balance and promoting overall scalp health.

To begin your journey toward a healthier scalp, start with a simple castor oil treatment. Warm a small amount of castor oil (about 2-4 tablespoons, depending on your hair length) in a microwave-safe bowl or a small pot. Be cautious not to overheat it; you want it warm enough to spread easily but not so hot that it burns your skin. Once it's at the right temperature, it's time to apply.

Using your fingertips, section your hair and gently massage the warm castor oil directly into your scalp. Focus on areas that feel dry or flaky, using circular motions to stimulate blood circulation. This massage not only helps distribute the oil evenly but also encourages the absorption of nutrients into the hair follicles. The soothing sensation will help relieve any itchiness associated with dandruff and leave your scalp feeling refreshed.

After massaging the oil in, let it sit for at least 30 minutes. For maximum benefits, consider wrapping your hair in a warm towel or using a shower cap. This will create a warm environment that allows the oil to penetrate deeper into the scalp. If you have time, leaving it on for a few hours or overnight can provide even more nourishment.

When you're ready to rinse, use a gentle, sulfate-free shampoo to cleanse your hair thoroughly. You may need to shampoo twice to ensure all the oil is removed. After washing, follow up with a light conditioner, focusing on the ends of your hair to avoid weighing down your roots.

In addition to this nourishing treatment, you can enhance the effectiveness of castor oil by blending it with other natural ingredients known for their scalp benefits. One popular combination is castor oil and tea tree oil. Tea tree oil is renowned for its antifungal and antibacterial properties, making it a powerful ally against dandruff. Mix a few drops of tea tree oil into your castor oil before application for an extra boost of scalp-clearing power.

Another great addition to your castor oil treatment is aloe vera gel. Aloe vera has soothing and moisturizing properties that can help alleviate scalp irritation and dryness. Combine equal parts of castor oil and aloe vera gel for a hydrating mask that not only nourishes the scalp but also promotes hair growth. Apply this mixture as you would with castor oil alone, massaging it in and allowing it to sit for at least 30 minutes before rinsing.

For those dealing with particularly stubborn dandruff or an irritated scalp, consider incorporating a gentle exfoliating scrub into your routine. You can create a simple homemade scrub using castor oil, sugar, and a few drops of your preferred essential oil for fragrance. Mix equal parts sugar and castor oil, then massage the scrub onto your scalp in circular motions. This will help remove dead skin cells and product buildup while keeping your scalp hydrated. Rinse thoroughly and follow up with your regular shampoo and conditioner.

To maintain a healthy scalp, it's essential to establish a regular routine. Aim to treat your scalp with castor oil once a week, gradually adjusting based on your scalp's response. If you notice significant improvement, you can reduce the frequency to every two weeks. Always listen to your body and adjust according to how your scalp feels.

In addition to topical treatments, remember that your diet plays a crucial role in scalp and hair health. Incorporate foods rich in vitamins A, C, D, and E, as well as omega-3 fatty acids, into your meals. These nutrients help support hair growth and maintain a healthy scalp. Staying hydrated is equally important—make sure you drink plenty of water throughout the day to keep your skin and scalp well-hydrated.

For those who prefer a more comprehensive approach, consider integrating castor oil into your lifestyle beyond topical applications. A daily dose of castor oil, either in a smoothie or taken directly, can also promote internal health and balance, benefiting your scalp and hair from the inside out. Just ensure to consult with a healthcare provider before incorporating it into your diet, especially if you have any existing health conditions.

Lastly, it's essential to recognize that patience is key. While castor oil can deliver impressive results, it won't work overnight. Consistency will lead to healthier hair and a flake-free scalp. Embrace the process, and enjoy the nourishing rituals as you watch your hair transform into a lively crown of beauty.

By harnessing the powerful properties of castor oil and integrating it into your hair care routine, you can effectively nourish your scalp, eliminate dandruff, and promote the growth of thick, healthy hair. With just a few simple steps, you are well on your way to achieving the luxurious locks you've always desired. So, embrace the golden oil and let its transformative powers elevate your hair care journey to new heights.

Creating luxurious hair masks with castor oil is a transformative experience that can revolutionize your hair care routine. This ancient oil, derived from the seeds of the Ricinus communis plant, has long been revered for its remarkable properties. Rich in ricinoleic acid, it not only nourishes and strengthens hair but also promotes healthy growth while preventing dryness and breakage. In this section, you'll discover how to create your own luxurious hair masks using castor oil, combining it with other natural ingredients to enhance its benefits and provide your hair with the pampering it deserves.

To start, let's explore the versatility of castor oil in hair masks. Its unique composition allows it to penetrate the hair shaft, delivering moisture deep within, which is essential for combating frizz and split ends. Additionally, castor oil can help improve scalp health by hydrating and soothing irritation, creating the perfect environment for hair to thrive.

When crafting your hair masks, consider your specific hair type and needs. Whether you have dry, oily, or normal hair, there's a combination that will work for you. Below are several recipes you can easily whip up at home, each designed to target different concerns while pampering your hair.

One of the most beneficial masks is the Castor Oil and Avocado Hair Mask. Avocado is known for its high fat content and vitamins A, D, and E, which nourish and strengthen hair. To prepare this mask, blend one ripe avocado with two tablespoons of castor oil until you achieve a smooth consistency. Apply the mixture to your hair from roots to tips, focusing on the ends where damage typically occurs. Leave the mask on for about 30-45 minutes, allowing the nutrients to penetrate deeply. Rinse thoroughly and follow up with your favorite shampoo and conditioner. This mask not only hydrates but also adds shine, leaving you with luscious, manageable hair.

If you're looking to boost hair growth, try the Castor Oil and Coconut Milk Hair Mask. Coconut milk is rich in proteins and essential fats that can help strengthen hair while adding moisture. To create this mask, combine three tablespoons of castor oil with half a cup of coconut milk in a bowl. Mix well and apply to your scalp and hair, massaging gently to stimulate circulation. Cover your hair with a shower cap, and let the mask sit for at least an hour before rinsing. This concoction not only smells divine but also nourishes your scalp, promoting healthy, faster hair growth.

For those battling dryness or brittleness, the Castor Oil and Honey Hair Mask is a must-try. Honey is a natural humectant that draws moisture into the hair, while castor oil seals it in. To make this mask, mix two tablespoons of castor oil with two tablespoons of raw honey. Apply it to damp hair, ensuring even distribution. Leave it on for 20-30 minutes before rinsing with warm water. The result is soft, hydrated hair that feels revitalized and looks healthy.

A more indulgent option is the Castor Oil and Essential Oil Hair Mask. Essential oils not only add a delightful aroma but can also provide additional benefits. For example, rosemary essential oil is known for its ability to stimulate hair growth, while lavender can soothe the scalp. To create this mask, mix two tablespoons of castor oil with a few drops of your chosen essential oil (around 5-10 drops). Apply this blend to your scalp and hair, gently massaging it in. Leave it on for up to an hour, allowing the essential oils to work their magic. Rinse thoroughly, and enjoy the calming scent and revitalized hair.

As you experiment with these masks, consider adding other nourishing ingredients to enhance their effectiveness. For instance, incorporating yogurt can add protein to your treatment, making it particularly effective for damaged hair. Simply mix one cup of plain yogurt with two tablespoons of castor oil and apply as you would with the other masks. The lactic acid in yogurt helps to exfoliate the scalp and remove buildup while conditioning the hair.

Another effective combination is the Castor Oil and Aloe Vera Hair Mask. Aloe vera is renowned for its soothing properties and is an excellent remedy for an irritated scalp. To create this mask, blend two tablespoons of castor oil with three tablespoons of fresh aloe vera gel. Apply it to your hair and scalp, focusing on areas that feel dry or itchy. Leave it on for 30-60 minutes before rinsing. This mask not only hydrates your hair but also promotes a healthier scalp environment.

When using these masks, don’t forget the importance of the application process. Before applying any mask, ensure your hair is clean and slightly damp for optimal absorption. Section your hair to make the application easier, and use a wide-tooth comb to distribute the mask evenly. After applying, consider wrapping your hair in a warm towel or using a shower cap to create a warming effect, which can enhance the mask's penetration.

Consistency is key to seeing results with any hair treatment. Aim to use these luxurious masks once a week for optimal benefits. As you incorporate castor oil into your hair care routine, you’ll likely notice improvements in texture, shine, and overall health.

Finally, remember that each person’s hair is unique, and it may take some experimentation to find the perfect combination for your specific needs. Keep a journal of your experiences, noting what works best for you. Over time, you'll develop a personalized hair mask regimen that enhances your hair's natural beauty.

Embrace the richness of castor oil and the power of nature as you indulge in these luxurious hair masks. With dedication and a little creativity, you’ll not only transform your hair but also discover a fulfilling and enjoyable self-care ritual that nourishes both your hair and spirit.

Chapter 4: Enhancing Brows and Lashes

For many, thick, well-defined eyebrows are synonymous with beauty and expression. They frame the face, enhance the eyes, and can even transform an entire look. However, factors such as over-plucking, genetics, and age can lead to sparse or thinning eyebrows. Fortunately, nature offers a remedy that has been cherished for centuries: castor oil. This potent oil, derived from the seeds of the castor bean plant, is rich in nutrients that nourish hair follicles, stimulate growth, and condition hair. If you're looking to thicken your eyebrows naturally, castor oil could be your answer.

One of the primary reasons castor oil is so effective for eyebrow enhancement lies in its composition. It contains a high concentration of ricinoleic acid, a unique fatty acid that promotes blood circulation to the hair follicles. This increased blood flow encourages hair growth by delivering essential nutrients and oxygen. Additionally, castor oil is packed with vitamin E, omega-6 and omega-9 fatty acids, and other nourishing compounds that strengthen hair strands, prevent breakage, and create a healthy environment for hair to thrive.

To start your journey toward fuller eyebrows, the first step is to source high-quality, cold-pressed castor oil. This method of extraction preserves the oil's natural properties, ensuring you receive the maximum benefits. Once you have your oil, you can easily incorporate it into your beauty routine.

Begin by cleansing your face thoroughly to remove any makeup or impurities. This allows the castor oil to penetrate deeply into the hair follicles without any barriers. Using a clean spoolie brush or a cotton swab, dip it into the castor oil and apply it directly to your eyebrows. Be generous, but avoid excess; you want to coat the hair and skin without dripping oil onto your face. As you apply, consider massaging the oil gently into your brows. This not only helps with absorption but also stimulates circulation, further enhancing growth potential.

For optimal results, allow the castor oil to sit on your eyebrows overnight. This gives the oil ample time to work its magic. If you prefer not to go to bed with oil on your face, you can leave it on for at least two hours before rinsing it off with lukewarm water. The key to success is consistency; aim to apply castor oil to your brows at least three to four times a week. Many users start noticing results within a few weeks, with fuller, thicker eyebrows becoming more apparent over time.

While castor oil is beneficial on its own, you can enhance its effects by mixing it with other natural ingredients known for promoting hair growth. For example, adding a few drops of essential oils such as rosemary or lavender can amplify the results. Rosemary oil, in particular, is celebrated for its ability to stimulate hair follicles and improve circulation, making it a perfect partner for castor oil. Combine one tablespoon of castor oil with a few drops of rosemary oil, mix well, and apply it to your brows using the same method described earlier.

Another effective combination involves using castor oil with almond oil, which is rich in vitamins and fatty acids that nourish and strengthen hair. Mixing equal parts of both oils creates a luxurious treatment that not only promotes growth but also conditions the hair, leaving your brows looking shiny and healthy. Apply this mixture as you would the castor oil alone for the best results.

If you find that the oil application feels too heavy or greasy, consider creating an eyebrow serum. Combine castor oil with aloe vera gel, which is known for its soothing properties and promotes hair growth. This gel-like consistency can make the application process easier and feel lighter on the skin. Simply mix one part castor oil with three parts aloe vera gel and apply it to your brows as you would normally.

In addition to topical treatments, maintaining a healthy diet can also contribute to eyebrow growth. Hair, including eyebrow hair, thrives on nutrients. Incorporate foods rich in vitamins A, C, E, and biotin, as well as omega fatty acids into your diet. Nuts, seeds, leafy greens, and fatty fish can provide the building blocks your body needs to support hair growth from the inside out.

It’s also crucial to be patient during your journey to thicker eyebrows. Hair growth takes time; on average, hair grows about half an inch per month. Avoid the temptation to pluck or shape your brows too frequently while you’re trying to enhance their fullness. Instead, let them grow out, and focus on nourishing them with castor oil and other beneficial ingredients.

Some individuals may experience irritation or allergic reactions to castor oil, so it’s wise to conduct a patch test before applying it directly to your eyebrows. Apply a small amount of oil to a discreet area of skin and wait 24 hours to see if any adverse reactions occur. If you experience redness, itching, or swelling, discontinue use.

As you embark on this journey to naturally thicken your eyebrows, remember that consistency and care are your best allies. Make castor oil a staple in your beauty routine, and be mindful of the other factors that contribute to healthy hair growth. With time, patience, and a little effort, you’ll find that your brows can transform from sparse to stunning, enhancing your natural beauty and giving you the confidence to embrace your unique look.

In the end, the art of achieving fuller eyebrows is not solely about the product you use, but also about the love and attention you give to your body. By harnessing the power of nature through castor oil, you're not just improving your appearance; you're embracing a holistic approach to beauty that celebrates health, wellness, and the beauty that comes from within. So go ahead, take that first step, and enjoy the transformation.

Eyelashes have long been celebrated as a symbol of beauty and femininity, framing the eyes and enhancing our expressions. While many of us turn to mascara or eyelash extensions to achieve that coveted volume, these methods can be costly and may even damage our natural lashes over time. Fortunately, castor oil offers a natural and effective solution for boosting eyelash volume, promoting not only length but also health and strength.

The secret to castor oil's effectiveness lies in its composition. Rich in ricinoleic acid, castor oil possesses anti-inflammatory and antimicrobial properties that can benefit the hair follicles. This oil is also packed with essential fatty acids, vitamin E, and proteins, all of which nourish and moisturize the hair, creating an optimal environment for growth. Regular use of castor oil on your eyelashes can lead to not just thicker lashes, but healthier ones, reducing the likelihood of breakage and promoting a fuller appearance.

To start, the application process is simple and requires minimal tools. You can use a clean mascara wand, an applicator brush, or even your fingertip. If using a mascara wand, ensure it's thoroughly cleaned to avoid any residue from previous products. Dip the wand into the castor oil and remove any excess oil to prevent drips. If you prefer using your fingertip, simply pour a small amount of castor oil into the palm of your hand and dip your finger in.

When applying castor oil, do so at night before bed. This allows ample time for the oil to penetrate the hair follicles while you sleep. Begin at the base of the eyelashes, applying the oil gently from the roots to the tips. Be careful to avoid getting the oil in your eyes, as it can cause irritation. If you do accidentally get some in your eyes, flush them with water. Not only does this process help in promoting lash growth, but it also conditions the lashes, making them appear glossier and more vibrant.

Consistency is key when it comes to using castor oil for eyelash enhancement. Aim for nightly application, making it a part of your bedtime routine. After a few weeks of regular use, you may start to notice subtle changes in your lashes. However, patience is essential; natural remedies work gradually, and results can take anywhere from four to six weeks to become visibly noticeable.

In addition to applying castor oil directly, consider combining it with other natural ingredients to amplify its effects. For instance, mixing castor oil with coconut oil can provide additional nourishment thanks to coconut oil's rich fatty acid content. This combination not only enhances lash health but also provides a delightful, soothing aroma during application. Alternatively, you can mix castor oil with vitamin E oil, which is renowned for its antioxidant properties that help combat free radicals, promoting healthier lashes over time.

Another fantastic option is to create a custom eyelash serum by combining castor oil with other essential oils known for their hair growth properties. Oils like rosemary, lavender, and peppermint have been shown to stimulate circulation and promote hair growth. Simply mix a few drops of your chosen essential oil with castor oil, and apply using the same method described earlier. Always conduct a patch test first to ensure you don't have any allergic reactions to these oils.

While castor oil is a fantastic tool for eyelash enhancement, maintaining the overall health of your lashes is equally important. Avoid harsh makeup removers that can strip the lashes of their natural oils. Opt for gentle, oil-based removers that will nourish rather than deplete the lashes. Furthermore, be cautious when applying mascara; opt for formulas that are free of harmful chemicals and parabens. Consider giving your lashes a break from mascara occasionally to allow them to breathe and recover.

Diet also plays a significant role in the health of your eyelashes. Ensure you are getting adequate nutrition by incorporating foods rich in vitamins and minerals essential for hair growth. Biotin, found in eggs, nuts, and whole grains, is particularly beneficial for hair health. Similarly, omega-3 fatty acids found in fish, flaxseeds, and walnuts can promote a healthy scalp and hair follicles, contributing to stronger lashes.

As you embark on this journey to boost your eyelash volume with castor oil, track your progress. Take before photos to compare your lashes over the weeks. You may be surprised by the transformation that occurs as your lashes become not only fuller but also healthier and more resilient. Engage with others in natural beauty communities or social media platforms where people share their experiences and tips with castor oil. There's a wealth of knowledge and support out there for those seeking to enhance their beauty through natural means.

Incorporating castor oil into your daily routine is more than just a beauty treatment; it's a self-care ritual that nurtures both your lashes and your spirit. As you pamper your lashes with this golden oil, you're also embracing a holistic approach to beauty that respects and celebrates your natural self. By choosing castor oil, you step away from the chemical-laden products that promise results but often deliver disappointment. Instead, you'll cultivate an authentic beauty that radiates from within, highlighting the eyes—the windows to your soul—with vibrant, luscious lashes that speak volumes.

To achieve the best results when enhancing your brows and lashes with castor oil, the application technique is just as critical as the oil itself. While castor oil is a powerhouse packed with nutrients and fatty acids that can promote hair growth and strengthen hair follicles, how you apply it can make a significant difference in the effectiveness of your treatments. Below, we'll explore a variety of methods to ensure you're getting the most out of your castor oil application.

The first step is to prepare your castor oil. Ideally, you want to use cold-pressed, organic castor oil, as this retains the most nutrients and ensures you're applying the purest form of the oil. If you want to enhance the oil further, consider mixing it with a few drops of essential oils like rosemary or lavender, which are known for their stimulating properties. However, be cautious with the quantities; a little goes a long way.

Before you begin the application, it's crucial to ensure that your brows and lashes are clean. Use a gentle cleanser to wash your face, removing any makeup, dirt, or oils that may be present. This will help the castor oil penetrate the hair follicles more effectively. Once your skin is clean, pat dry gently with a towel.

For brow application, you can use a clean mascara wand or a cotton swab. If you opt for the mascara wand, ensure it's freshly washed and free of any old product. Dip the wand into the castor oil, allowing any excess to drip off. Carefully apply the oil to your eyebrows by brushing it in the direction of hair growth. Focus on the areas where your brows are sparse or thinner. The gentle massaging action of the wand will not only distribute the oil but also stimulate blood circulation in the area, promoting growth.

If you prefer using a cotton swab, dip one end into the castor oil, then gently apply it to your brows using small strokes. This method allows for precision and is especially effective for targeting specific areas. Again, make sure to massage the oil into your skin and brow hairs, as this can enhance absorption.

For eyelash application, you can use a clean eyeliner brush or the same mascara wand you used for your brows. The process is quite similar. Dip the brush into the castor oil, and carefully apply it to your lashes, starting from the roots and working your way to the tips. Be cautious not to use too much oil, as it can get into your eyes and cause irritation. Only a thin layer is necessary to reap the benefits.

Another method for lash application is to use your fingertip. Put a small amount of castor oil on your fingertip and gently apply it to your lashes. This method can feel more natural and allows for a more tactile application, helping you to sense how much product you’re using and where you're applying it.

One of the most effective techniques for both brows and lashes is to apply the castor oil before bedtime. The oil needs time to work, and leaving it on overnight allows for maximum absorption and effectiveness. After applying the oil, you can go to sleep without worrying about smudging or removing it until morning. Just be cautious if you tend to rub your eyes in your sleep; consider using a clean cloth or placing a towel over your pillow to avoid any potential mess.

Consistency is key when using castor oil for brow and lash enhancement. Aim to apply the oil at least 3-4 times a week for optimal results. Track your progress by taking before and after photos every few weeks. This not only helps you see the changes but also keeps you motivated to stick with your routine.

While you may start to see results in just a few weeks, full results can take a couple of months, as hair growth is a gradual process. Patience is essential here, as your brows and lashes may need time to absorb the nutrients and grow stronger. During this time, you may also want to evaluate your overall health and diet, as these can play significant roles in hair growth. Incorporating foods rich in vitamins A, C, E, and omega-3 fatty acids can support your brow and lash health from the inside out.

Finally, remember that while castor oil is a natural remedy, individual results may vary. Some people may notice significant improvements in the density and strength of their brows and lashes, while others may experience more subtle changes. It's also essential to be mindful of any allergic reactions. If you notice any redness, itching, or swelling, discontinue use immediately and consult with a healthcare professional.

By following these application techniques and maintaining a consistent routine, you're setting yourself up for success in your journey to enhance your brows and lashes naturally. With the power of castor oil, you can achieve fuller, healthier eyebrows and eyelashes that not only frame your face beautifully but also contribute to your overall confidence and appearance. As you embark on this self-care ritual, take a moment to enjoy the process and celebrate the natural beauty of your brows and lashes.

Chapter 5: Complete Body Care

Creating your own luxurious body lotions with castor oil is not only a rewarding experience but also an effective way to pamper your skin with natural goodness. Castor oil, known for its rich essential fatty acids, is a powerful moisturizer that deeply penetrates the skin, providing hydration and nourishment. By blending it with other natural oils and ingredients, you can craft personalized lotions that cater to your skin's unique needs, leaving it soft, supple, and radiant.

To embark on this journey of self-care, let's explore various formulations and techniques that will empower you to create body lotions tailored to your preferences. The key is to combine castor oil with carriers, essential oils, and other beneficial ingredients that enhance its properties while providing delightful scents and textures.

One popular base for body lotions is a blend of carrier oils, which serve to dilute the potency of castor oil while enhancing the lotion's overall consistency. Sweet almond oil, coconut oil, and jojoba oil are excellent choices. Sweet almond oil is particularly beneficial for dry skin due to its emollient properties, while coconut oil adds a delightful tropical fragrance and offers antibacterial benefits. Jojoba oil is closely related to the skin's natural sebum, making it perfect for all skin types.

To begin creating your luxurious body lotion, start with a simple recipe as a foundation. In a double boiler, combine half a cup of castor oil with half a cup of your chosen carrier oil. Heat gently until the oils are fully melted and blended. This base will serve as the foundation of your lotion, delivering deep hydration.

Once you have your oil mixture, it's time to add a few drops of essential oils for fragrance and additional skin benefits. Lavender essential oil is renowned for its calming properties and can help soothe irritated skin, while tea tree oil is excellent for its antimicrobial effects, making it ideal for acne-prone skin. For a refreshing scent, consider peppermint or eucalyptus oil, which can invigorate the senses and provide a cooling sensation when applied.

After adding your essential oils, it's beneficial to incorporate natural butters into your body lotion. Shea butter and cocoa butter are both superb options that enhance the creamy texture of your lotion while providing an extra layer of hydration. Adding a quarter cup of shea butter to your oil mixture can enrich your lotion, making it perfect for particularly dry areas such as elbows and knees.

To achieve the desired consistency, you may want to thicken your lotion further. This can be done by adding beeswax to the oil mixture. Beeswax acts as a natural emulsifier, helping to bind the oils and butters together. Add about two tablespoons of grated beeswax to your mixture and allow it to melt completely. Once melted, remove the mixture from heat and let it cool slightly.

At this point, the lotion can be transferred to a blender or mixer for a fluffier texture. Blend the oil and wax mixture for a minute or two, allowing it to cool further and become airy. This step can enhance the feel of your lotion, making it luxurious and light yet intensely hydrating.

Once you're satisfied with the consistency, pour your body lotion into clean, sterilized jars or bottles. Allow the lotion to cool completely before sealing the containers. To personalize your creations, consider labeling them with the date and the specific blend of essential oils you used, so you can replicate your favorites in the future.

As you experiment with these formulations, you can also explore additional ingredients that promote skin health. For instance, vitamin E oil acts as a powerful antioxidant that can help prolong the shelf life of your lotion while nourishing the skin. Adding a teaspoon of vitamin E oil to your mixture can provide extra moisture and protection.

Another exciting ingredient to consider is aloe vera gel, which can enhance hydration and soothe irritated skin. If you choose to incorporate aloe vera, mix it in after blending your oils and butters, and use it immediately, as it does not have a long shelf life.

Creating your own body lotion with castor oil allows you to express your creativity while harnessing the benefits of nature. The process can be a therapeutic ritual, offering you a moment of mindfulness and self-care. It's a chance to connect with the ingredients you're using, understanding their properties and how they benefit your skin.

When using your homemade lotion, apply it generously after a shower or bath when your skin is still damp. This practice locks in moisture and enhances the lotion's hydrating effects. For a luxurious experience, consider taking a few moments to massage the lotion into your skin, promoting circulation and relaxation.

As you delve into the world of body care with castor oil, remember that the journey is as important as the destination. Each formulation you create is an opportunity to learn about your skin's needs, discover new scents and textures, and embrace a more natural and holistic approach to beauty.

With the knowledge and recipes shared, you can transform your self-care routines through the creation of luxurious body lotions that hydrate, nourish, and pamper your skin. Castor oil, with its rich history and proven benefits, serves as the perfect cornerstone for your body care rituals, allowing you to cultivate a glowing, healthy complexion naturally. Embrace the power of self-made beauty, and let your skin thrive with the nourishing touch of castor oil.

Exfoliating scrubs are essential tools in the quest for smooth, glowing skin. By removing dead skin cells, they not only reveal a fresher layer beneath but also allow for better absorption of moisturizers and other skincare products. Castor oil, with its unique properties, serves as a powerful base for these scrubs, enhancing their effectiveness while nourishing the skin.

When creating an exfoliating scrub with castor oil, you benefit from the oil's high ricinoleic acid content, which possesses anti-inflammatory and antibacterial properties. This makes it an excellent choice for soothing irritated skin and fighting acne-causing bacteria. Additionally, castor oil is rich in fatty acids, which help to hydrate and protect the skin, preventing dryness that can often accompany exfoliation.

To craft a simple yet effective exfoliating scrub, you can start with a base of natural exfoliants. Common choices include sugar, salt, and ground coffee. Each of these has unique properties: sugar is gentle and perfect for sensitive skin, salt offers a more vigorous exfoliation suitable for tougher areas like elbows and knees, while coffee grounds not only exfoliate but also stimulate blood circulation, giving your skin a vibrant glow.

Here’s a recipe to get you started on your journey to smoother skin:

Castor Oil and Sugar Exfoliating Scrub

Ingredients: - 1 cup granulated sugar (white or brown) - 1/2 cup castor oil - 1 teaspoon vanilla extract (optional, for fragrance) - A few drops of your favorite essential oil (optional)

Instructions: 1. In a mixing bowl, combine the granulated sugar and castor oil. Mix well until the sugar is fully coated in the oil. 2. If you're using it, add the vanilla extract and essential oil, stirring until evenly distributed. 3. Transfer the mixture into an airtight container. This scrub can be stored for up to two weeks.

When using your scrub, dampen your skin in the shower or bath. Take a handful of the scrub and gently massage it onto your skin in circular motions, focusing on dry or rough areas. Rinse off with warm water and pat your skin dry. The result? Silky-smooth skin that feels rejuvenated and refreshed.

For those who prefer a salt-based scrub, you can follow a similar recipe. However, keep in mind that salt can be a bit more abrasive, so it may not be suitable for sensitive skin types. If you're dealing with body acne or rough patches, though, a salt scrub could be just what you need.

Castor Oil and Salt Exfoliating Scrub

Ingredients: - 1 cup coarse sea salt (or Himalayan salt) - 1/2 cup castor oil - Zest from one lemon or lime (for a refreshing scent and additional skin benefits) - A few drops of tea tree oil (known for its antibacterial properties)

Instructions: 1. Combine the salt and castor oil in a bowl, mixing until the salt is well coated. 2. Add the citrus zest and tea tree oil, stirring to combine. 3. Store in an airtight container, and use within two weeks for the best results.

The addition of citrus zest not only enhances the scrub's scent but also provides a dose of antioxidants and natural brightening properties. This can help to even out skin tone and reduce the appearance of dark spots over time.

Another option is a coffee-based scrub, which makes for a great morning ritual thanks to its invigorating scent and energizing qualities. Coffee scrubs are known for their ability to help reduce the appearance of cellulite and promote circulation, giving the skin a firm, youthful appearance.

Castor Oil and Coffee Scrub

Ingredients: - 1 cup ground coffee - 1/2 cup castor oil - 1/4 cup brown sugar (to add a gentle exfoliating touch) - A few drops of peppermint essential oil (for a refreshing tingle)

Instructions: 1. In a bowl, mix together the ground coffee, castor oil, and brown sugar until well combined. 2. Add the peppermint oil and mix again. 3. Store in an airtight container, and use within two weeks.

To use, apply the scrub to damp skin just like the previous scrubs, massaging in circular motions. Rinse well, and enjoy the invigorating aroma and smooth texture that lingers on your skin.

While exfoliating scrubs can work wonders for your skin, it's essential to remember that moderation is key. Over-exfoliating can lead to irritation, redness, and even breakouts. Aim to exfoliate 1-2 times a week, depending on your skin type. Those with oily skin may benefit from more frequent exfoliation, while those with dry or sensitive skin should stick to less frequent applications.

After using an exfoliating scrub, it’s vital to follow up with a good moisturizer. Castor oil itself can be used as a post-exfoliation treatment, as it will help lock in moisture and provide a protective barrier against environmental stressors. Simply massage a small amount of castor oil into your skin to maintain its smoothness and hydration.

You might also want to experiment with different combinations and additions to your scrubs. For instance, incorporating honey can provide additional antibacterial benefits, while oatmeal can add a soothing element for irritated skin. The possibilities are endless, and you can tailor your scrubs to meet your skin's specific needs.

As you delve into the world of exfoliating scrubs with castor oil, remember that the journey to smooth skin is not just about the products you use; it’s also about self-care and taking the time to pamper yourself. Making these scrubs can transform your skincare routine into a delightful ritual, allowing you to connect with your body and appreciate the results of your efforts. Embrace the process, enjoy the journey, and watch your skin flourish with the nourishing power of castor oil.

Scars, whether from acne, injuries, or surgeries, can serve as a constant reminder of past experiences. Many people feel self-conscious about their scars, leading them to seek out solutions that promise to diminish their appearance. While there are countless products on the market with aggressive chemical formulations, nature offers a gentler, more effective alternative: castor oil.

Rich in ricinoleic acid, castor oil has powerful anti-inflammatory properties that can help reduce the redness and swelling associated with scars. This unique oil promotes the regeneration of skin tissues, making it a go-to remedy for fading scars and improving overall skin texture. Furthermore, castor oil’s thick consistency ensures that it adheres well to the skin, allowing for prolonged absorption and enhanced efficacy.

To harness the scar-fading potential of castor oil, you can create simple yet effective treatments at home. Below are a few recipes and application techniques designed to help you achieve smoother, more even-toned skin.

One of the simplest methods involves using pure castor oil directly on the scarred area. To do this, start with clean, dry skin. Apply a small amount of castor oil onto your fingertips or a cotton pad and gently massage it into the scar for about 5 to 10 minutes. This helps increase blood circulation to the area, promoting healing and reducing the appearance of the scar. For best results, consider doing this twice a day—once in the morning and once before bed.

For those looking to enhance the benefits of castor oil, combining it with other natural ingredients can create a powerful scar-fading treatment. One such combination is castor oil with vitamin E oil. Vitamin E is renowned for its skin-healing properties and can significantly improve the appearance of scars. To create this treatment, mix equal parts of castor oil and vitamin E oil in a small bowl. Use the same massage technique as before, applying the mixture to the scarred area and working it into the skin. The antioxidant properties of vitamin E can help repair damaged skin while the ricinoleic acid in castor oil facilitates new cell growth.

Another effective recipe involves adding essential oils that have scar-fading properties. Lavender essential oil, for example, is known for its soothing qualities and ability to promote skin regeneration. To create a nourishing blend, combine two tablespoons of castor oil with 5 to 10 drops of lavender essential oil. Apply this mixture as you would the pure castor oil, massaging it into the scarred area. The calming scent of lavender also provides a relaxing experience, making it an excellent addition to your skincare routine.

If you're dealing with larger scars or stretch marks, creating a castor oil pack can be particularly beneficial. A castor oil pack involves soaking a piece of flannel or cotton cloth in castor oil and applying it to the affected area. To make the pack, saturate a piece of cloth with castor oil, then place it over the scar. To enhance absorption, cover the cloth with plastic wrap, and apply a heating pad or hot water bottle over the area for 30 to 60 minutes. The heat helps the oil penetrate deeper into the skin, promoting healing and reducing the appearance of scars over time. This method can be done several times a week for optimal results.

For those who enjoy incorporating natural ingredients into their skincare routine, consider making a castor oil scrub. Combining castor oil with sugar or coffee grounds creates an exfoliating treatment that helps remove dead skin cells, allowing healthier skin to surface. To prepare this scrub, mix two tablespoons of castor oil with one tablespoon of sugar or coffee grounds. In the shower or bath, gently massage the scrub onto the scarred area in circular motions, then rinse thoroughly. This not only helps fade scars but also leaves your skin feeling soft and refreshed.

Hydration is essential for scar healing, and mixing castor oil with aloe vera can boost hydration while providing soothing relief. Aloe vera is known for its healing properties and is often used to treat burns and skin irritations. To create a healing gel, combine two tablespoons of castor oil with two tablespoons of fresh aloe vera gel. Apply this mixture to the scarred area and let it sit for 20 minutes before rinsing. This combination not only helps to fade scars but also deeply moisturizes and soothes the skin.

While these treatments can be incredibly effective, consistency is key. Scars often take time to fade, and maintaining a regular routine will yield the best results. Keep in mind that individual results may vary based on skin type, age, and the severity of the scars. It's also essential to perform a patch test before applying any new treatment to ensure your skin does not react negatively.

Lastly, remember that while castor oil is a powerful ally in your journey toward scar reduction, it works best when combined with a holistic approach to skincare. Staying hydrated, eating a balanced diet rich in vitamins and minerals, and protecting your skin from sun exposure can all contribute to healthier skin and more effective scar healing.

Incorporating castor oil into your scar management routine empowers you with a natural solution that aligns with your wellness goals. With a little patience and dedication, you can diminish the appearance of scars and unveil smoother, more radiant skin. The journey to recovery may take time, but with each application, you are taking a step toward embracing your skin's natural beauty.

Chapter 6: Pain and Inflammation Relief

Joint pain can be a debilitating condition that affects people of all ages and lifestyles. Whether it's due to arthritis, overuse, or injury, finding effective relief is a top priority for many. Traditional pharmaceuticals often come with a host of side effects, leading many individuals to seek out natural alternatives. Fortunately, castor oil has emerged as a powerful ally in the fight against joint pain and inflammation, thanks to its unique properties and beneficial compounds.

The primary component of castor oil, ricinoleic acid, is known for its anti-inflammatory effects. This fatty acid interacts with the body's pain receptors, helping to reduce inflammation and alleviate discomfort. When applied topically, castor oil penetrates the skin quickly, delivering its soothing properties directly to the affected area. This not only provides relief but also promotes overall joint health.

To get started with using castor oil for joint pain relief, consider a simple massage technique that can be both therapeutic and relaxing. Begin by warming a small amount of castor oil in the palm of your hands. The warmth will enhance the oil's absorption and effectiveness. Once the oil is warmed, gently massage it into the painful area using circular motions. This not only helps the oil penetrate the skin but also increases blood flow to the area, further aiding in pain relief.

For added efficacy, consider combining castor oil with other natural ingredients known for their anti-inflammatory properties. For example, mixing castor oil with essential oils such as eucalyptus or peppermint can create a potent pain-relieving blend.

Eucalyptus oil is known for its cooling sensation and ability to reduce pain and swelling, while peppermint oil has a calming effect that can ease muscle tension. To create this blend, mix two tablespoons of castor oil with a few drops of your chosen essential oil, then massage the mixture into your joints.

Another effective approach is to use castor oil as part of a warm compress. To prepare a warm compress, soak a clean cloth in warm castor oil, then wring it out to remove excess oil. Place the cloth on the affected joint and cover it with plastic wrap to retain heat. The warmth will enhance the oil's absorption, allowing its anti-inflammatory properties to work more effectively. Leave the compress on for 30 minutes to an hour, giving your body time to absorb the beneficial compounds.

In addition to topical applications, incorporating castor oil into your diet can also support joint health from the inside out. Consuming castor oil can promote digestive health and reduce inflammation throughout the body. However, it’s essential to use castor oil in moderation and consult with a healthcare professional before making any significant changes to your diet.

For those looking to further enhance the benefits of castor oil, consider engaging in gentle exercises that promote joint mobility. Activities such as yoga and swimming can help improve flexibility and strength without putting excessive strain on your joints. When combined with castor oil treatments, these exercises can help build a comprehensive approach to joint health.

In addition to its anti-inflammatory properties, castor oil is also known for its ability to promote blood circulation. Improved circulation can help deliver oxygen and nutrients to the joints, further supporting their health. To take advantage of this benefit, consider incorporating castor oil into your daily self-care routine.

A great way to do this is by creating a soothing castor oil bath soak. Simply add a few tablespoons of castor oil to your warm bath water. The warmth of the water helps to open your pores and allows the oil to penetrate your skin more effectively. Soaking in the bath can not only provide relief to sore joints but also promote relaxation and stress relief, which can be beneficial for managing pain.

As with any natural remedy, consistency is key. Regularly incorporating castor oil into your joint pain relief routine can yield better results over time. Keep a journal to track your progress, noting any changes in pain levels, mobility, or overall wellbeing. This will not only help you stay motivated but also allow you to identify which treatments work best for you.

While castor oil can be incredibly beneficial for joint pain relief, it's essential to listen to your body. If you experience increased pain or discomfort after using castor oil, discontinue use and consult a healthcare professional. Additionally, castor oil should not be used on open wounds or broken skin, as it may cause irritation.

In summary, castor oil offers a natural and effective approach to alleviating joint pain and inflammation. Its anti-inflammatory properties, combined with its ability to enhance circulation, make it a powerful ally in promoting joint health. By incorporating castor oil into your daily routine through massage, warm compresses, or even a soothing bath, you can take significant strides toward reducing pain and improving your overall quality of life. As with any natural remedy, patience and consistency are essential, so give yourself time to experience the full benefits of this golden oil. Embrace the power of castor oil, and take control of your joint health today.

Muscle aches can be a frustrating and debilitating experience, often impacting your ability to perform daily activities or enjoy your favorite hobbies. Whether it's the result of an intense workout, poor posture, or simply the wear and tear of everyday life, muscle soreness can leave you feeling drained and uncomfortable. Fortunately, castor oil offers a natural, effective solution to help alleviate these aches and promote recovery.

Rich in ricinoleic acid, castor oil possesses remarkable anti-inflammatory properties that can significantly reduce muscle pain and inflammation. When applied topically, this golden oil penetrates the skin, delivering its healing benefits directly to the affected area. Unlike over-the-counter pain relievers that may come with unwanted side effects, castor oil offers a gentle yet powerful alternative that aligns with your body's natural healing processes.

To maximize the benefits of castor oil for muscle aches, consider incorporating it into your post-exercise routine or as a part of your self-care regimen. One effective method is to create a warming castor oil compress. Start by heating a small amount of castor oil in a double boiler or microwave until it reaches a comfortable temperature—be sure it's not too hot to avoid burns. Soak a clean cloth in the warmed oil, wring it out, and place it over the sore muscle. Cover the cloth with a heating pad or a hot water bottle to enhance absorption. This method not only helps to soothe the aching muscle but also promotes circulation, which can aid in the healing process.

Another way to harness the power of castor oil is through massage. Mixing castor oil with a carrier oil, such as coconut or olive oil, can create a luxurious and soothing massage oil. The combination of gentle pressure and castor oil can help relax tense muscles and stimulate blood flow to the area, facilitating recovery. As you massage the oil into the sore muscles, focus on using steady, firm strokes. This not only enhances the effectiveness of the treatment but also provides a calming experience, helping to alleviate any stress or tension that may be exacerbating your discomfort.

For those who prefer a more hands-off approach, consider adding castor oil to your bath routine. Simply mix a few tablespoons of castor oil into your warm bathwater, allowing your muscles to soak in its therapeutic properties. The warmth of the water will open your pores, enabling the castor oil to penetrate deeper into your skin for maximum benefit. This method is particularly effective for widespread muscle aches, as it allows for full-body relaxation and revitalization.

In addition to topical applications, castor oil can also support muscle recovery from within. Incorporating castor oil into your diet can provide systemic benefits that promote overall wellness. A tablespoon of castor oil, taken internally, can help to reduce inflammation throughout the body. However, it's essential to consult with a healthcare professional before consuming castor oil, especially if you are new to it or have any underlying health conditions.

As you explore the myriad ways to use castor oil for muscle relief, remember that consistency is key. Integrating this natural remedy into your routine can lead to cumulative benefits, helping to manage muscle aches effectively over time. To support the healing process, also consider complementing your castor oil treatments with other holistic practices, such as gentle stretching, yoga, or low-impact exercises. These activities can help maintain flexibility and strength, reducing the risk of future muscle soreness.

It's also essential to listen to your body. If you experience persistent or severe muscle pain, it's advisable to consult a healthcare professional. While castor oil can provide relief for many common aches and pains, understanding the underlying cause of your discomfort is crucial for effective treatment and prevention.

In addition to its anti-inflammatory properties, castor oil is rich in antioxidants, which can help combat oxidative stress in the body. This makes it a valuable ally not only in managing muscle aches but also in supporting overall muscle health. By addressing inflammation and promoting recovery, castor oil aids in maintaining the integrity of muscle tissue, which is essential for optimal physical performance.

Many individuals have reported positive experiences using castor oil for muscle relief, with countless testimonials highlighting its effectiveness. From athletes seeking faster recovery times to individuals with chronic pain, the versatility of castor oil has made it a beloved natural remedy across various demographics. By sharing your experiences and incorporating castor oil into your wellness practices, you may inspire others to explore its benefits.

As you delve into the world of muscle care with castor oil, don't shy away from experimenting with different methods and combinations. Each body is unique, and what works best for you may vary. Keep track of your experiences and remain open to discovering new ways to incorporate this powerful oil into your pain management routine.

Ultimately, the journey towards relief from muscle aches is not just about finding a remedy; it's about embracing a holistic approach to well-being. By integrating castor oil into your self-care practices, you can empower your body to heal itself, promoting not only muscle recovery but also overall vitality. As you embark on this path, remember that healing takes time, and nurturing your body with natural solutions can lead to lasting benefits that extend well beyond alleviating pain. With patience and persistence, castor oil can become a trusted ally in your quest for a healthier, more resilient you.

Inflammation is the body's natural response to injury or infection, acting as a protective mechanism to promote healing. However, when inflammation becomes chronic, it can lead to a myriad of health issues, including pain, fatigue, and even more serious conditions like arthritis, heart disease, and diabetes. Many people turn to pharmaceuticals for relief, but these often come with unwanted side effects and can sometimes mask the underlying issues instead of addressing them. Fortunately, castor oil offers a natural alternative to reduce inflammation and promote healing without the risks associated with conventional medications.

The key to castor oil's effectiveness in reducing inflammation lies in its unique composition. It is rich in ricinoleic acid, a fatty acid known for its anti-inflammatory properties. Studies have shown that ricinoleic acid can inhibit the production of certain pro-inflammatory cytokines, which are signaling molecules that play a crucial role in the inflammatory process. By incorporating castor oil into your wellness routine, you can harness its healing potential to alleviate pain and reduce inflammation in a safe, natural way.

One of the most popular methods to use castor oil for inflammation is through topical application. The oil can be massaged directly onto the affected area, where it penetrates the skin and interacts with immune cells to reduce swelling and discomfort. For optimal results, warm the oil slightly before application. This can enhance absorption and provide additional relief through the soothing warmth against sore muscles or joints.

To create an effective anti-inflammatory treatment, consider blending castor oil with essential oils known for their healing properties. For instance, adding a few drops of peppermint or eucalyptus oil can enhance the cooling effect and provide pain relief, while lavender oil promotes relaxation and a sense of calm. Combine two tablespoons of castor oil with a few drops of your chosen essential oils, then gently massage the mixture into the affected area. This blend not only targets inflammation but also creates a nurturing self-care ritual that can help alleviate stress and promote overall well-being.

Another powerful way to utilize castor oil is through a technique called castor oil packs. This method has been used for centuries and is particularly effective for larger areas of inflammation, such as the abdomen or back. To create a castor oil pack, you'll need a piece of flannel or cotton cloth, castor oil, plastic wrap, and a heating pad or hot water bottle.

Start by saturating the cloth with castor oil, ensuring it's thoroughly soaked but not dripping. Place the cloth directly on the area of inflammation, then cover it with plastic wrap to prevent any mess. Finally, apply a heating pad or hot water bottle over the pack to help the oil penetrate the skin more deeply. Aim to leave the pack on for at least 30 minutes, allowing the oil to work its magic. This method can be particularly beneficial for conditions like arthritis or chronic pain, as it not only reduces inflammation but also promotes blood circulation and enhances the overall healing process.

In addition to topical applications, castor oil can also be ingested to help reduce internal inflammation. When consuming castor oil, it's crucial to do so in moderation, as it is a potent laxative. Starting with half a teaspoon per day is often recommended, gradually increasing the dosage if needed. Some people prefer to mix castor oil with a small amount of honey or juice to mask its strong taste. This internal use may help reduce inflammation in the digestive tract, alleviating symptoms of conditions like irritable bowel syndrome (IBS) and promoting overall gut health.

For those looking to support their body's inflammatory response through diet, complementing the use of castor oil with anti-inflammatory foods can enhance the effects. Incorporate a variety of colorful fruits and vegetables, healthy fats like olive oil and avocados, and omega-3-rich foods such as fatty fish and flaxseeds into your meals. These foods contain antioxidants and other compounds that work synergistically with castor oil to combat inflammation and promote healing.

Exercise is another vital component of reducing inflammation naturally. Gentle activities such as yoga, walking, or swimming can help improve circulation, reduce stress, and promote the release of endorphins, which are natural pain relievers produced by the body. When combined with the soothing properties of castor oil, regular movement can significantly improve your overall well-being and resilience against inflammation.

While castor oil is an excellent natural remedy for inflammation, it's essential to approach your health holistically. This means paying attention to your lifestyle, stress levels, and dietary choices. Reducing stress through mindfulness practices, like meditation or deep breathing exercises, can also contribute to decreased inflammation in the body. When combined with the anti-inflammatory benefits of castor oil, you create a powerful toolkit for managing pain and fostering overall health.

It's important to note that while many individuals experience positive results from using castor oil, everyone's body is different. Start with small applications and listen to your body’s responses. If you have any pre-existing conditions or are on medication, consult with a healthcare professional before beginning any new treatment regimen, including natural remedies like castor oil.

In conclusion, reducing inflammation without pharmaceuticals is not only possible but can be effectively achieved through the use of castor oil. By leveraging its anti-inflammatory properties through topical applications, castor oil packs, and even internal consumption, you can address pain and discomfort naturally. Coupled with a balanced diet, regular exercise, and mindful practices, castor oil can be a cornerstone of your journey towards better health and wellness. Embrace this golden oil and unlock the potential for a life free from the burden of chronic inflammation.

Chapter 7: Women's Health Remedies

Cellulite and stretch marks are two common concerns that many women face, often leading to feelings of insecurity and frustration. While they are entirely normal physiological occurrences, the desire to reduce their visibility is perfectly understandable. Fortunately, castor oil can be a powerful ally in your journey toward smoother skin and greater confidence.

Cellulite, characterized by dimpled skin, occurs when fat deposits push through the connective tissue beneath the skin, creating that bumpy appearance. This condition is influenced by a variety of factors, including genetics, hormonal changes, and lifestyle choices. Stretch marks, on the other hand, are streaks or lines that appear when the skin stretches or shrinks rapidly, often due to weight fluctuations, pregnancy, or puberty. While these marks are harmless, they can be a source of distress for many women.

The good news is that castor oil, with its rich composition of fatty acids and anti-inflammatory properties, can help improve the appearance of both cellulite and stretch marks. By incorporating castor oil into your skincare routine, you can take proactive steps toward enhancing your skin's elasticity, promoting healing, and reducing the appearance of these common concerns.

One of the primary benefits of castor oil is its high ricinoleic acid content. This unique fatty acid has been shown to improve blood circulation and lymphatic drainage, which can help in reducing the appearance of cellulite. When applied topically, castor oil penetrates deeply into the skin, providing hydration and nourishment while promoting skin elasticity. This is essential, as well-hydrated skin is more resilient and less likely to succumb to the formation of stretch marks.

To use castor oil for reducing cellulite, start by preparing your skin. Gently exfoliate the area with a homemade scrub made from sugar and a few drops of castor oil. This will help remove dead skin cells, allowing the oil to penetrate more effectively. After exfoliating, apply a generous amount of castor oil to the affected areas, massaging it in with firm, circular motions. This massage not only helps the oil absorb but also stimulates circulation, further aiding in the breakdown of fat deposits that contribute to cellulite.

For added benefits, consider mixing castor oil with other essential oils known for their skin-tightening and firming properties. Essential oils such as grapefruit, juniper, and rosemary are excellent choices. Simply blend a few drops of your chosen essential oil with castor oil before application. This not only enhances the effectiveness of your treatment but also leaves your skin smelling delightful.

In addition to topical application, maintaining a healthy lifestyle is crucial for managing cellulite. Regular exercise, particularly strength training and cardiovascular workouts, can help tone the muscles and reduce fat accumulation beneath the skin. Staying hydrated and consuming a balanced diet rich in antioxidants, healthy fats, and fiber will also support your skin's health, helping to prevent the formation of new stretch marks and cellulite.

Now, let's shift our focus to stretch marks. While it's impossible to completely eliminate them, castor oil can significantly diminish their appearance, especially if used during their initial formation stages. The moisturizing properties of castor oil keep the skin supple, which is essential during times of rapid change, such as pregnancy or weight loss. By applying castor oil to areas prone to stretch marks—like the abdomen, thighs, and breasts—you can help maintain skin elasticity and reduce the likelihood of these marks forming.

For optimal results, apply castor oil daily to the areas of concern. You may also want to consider creating a nourishing blend by adding vitamin E oil or aloe vera gel to your castor oil. Vitamin E is known for its skin-healing properties and can help improve skin texture, while aloe vera enhances hydration and soothes any irritation. Simply mix equal parts of castor oil and your chosen additive, then massage the mixture into your skin in gentle, circular motions.

Consistency is key when it comes to treating both cellulite and stretch marks. By making castor oil a part of your daily routine, you're not just targeting the appearance of these concerns; you're also nurturing your skin from within. Keep in mind that results may take time, and every individual's skin responds differently, so be patient and stay committed to your regimen.

In addition to topical treatments, you may also want to explore some lifestyle changes that can further support your skin's health. Incorporating foods high in antioxidants, such as berries, leafy greens, and nuts, can help combat oxidative stress, which may contribute to skin aging and the formation of stretch marks. Staying hydrated by drinking plenty of water will keep your skin plump and elastic, making it less susceptible to damage.

Lastly, consider practicing mindfulness and stress management techniques. Stress can lead to hormonal fluctuations that may exacerbate skin issues, including cellulite and stretch marks. Engaging in activities such as yoga, meditation, or even simple breathing exercises can help you cultivate a sense of calm and balance, contributing positively to your overall well-being and skin health.

With dedication and the right approach, you can effectively reduce the appearance of cellulite and stretch marks using castor oil as a natural remedy. Empower yourself by embracing this age-old solution, and take pride in nurturing your skin naturally. Remember, your body is a testament to your unique journey, and every mark tells a story. With castor oil as your ally, you can enhance your confidence and embrace your beauty, inside and out.

Menstrual cramps, or dysmenorrhea, are a common experience for many women, often bringing discomfort that can significantly affect daily life. While the menstrual cycle is a natural process, the pain associated with it can vary in intensity and duration, leaving many searching for effective remedies. In this pursuit, castor oil emerges as a powerful ally, offering natural relief without the side effects often associated with over-the-counter medications.

Understanding how castor oil can alleviate menstrual cramps starts with its unique composition. This oil is rich in ricinoleic acid, a compound known for its anti-inflammatory and analgesic properties. When applied topically, castor oil penetrates the skin and interacts with receptors that help reduce pain and inflammation. This quality makes castor oil particularly effective for treating the discomfort associated with menstrual cramps.

To harness the benefits of castor oil for menstrual pain, you can create a simple yet effective castor oil pack. This method not only delivers the oil's healing properties directly to the affected area but also promotes relaxation and comfort. Here’s how you can make and use a castor oil pack:

1. Gather Your Supplies: You'll need a piece of flannel or cotton cloth, castor oil, plastic wrap, and a heating pad or hot water bottle.

2. Prepare the Pack: Soak the cloth in castor oil until it is saturated but not dripping. Place the cloth on your lower abdomen, where you typically feel the cramps.

3. Cover and Heat: Wrap the soaked cloth with plastic wrap to avoid any mess and place a heating pad or hot water bottle on top. The warmth will enhance the oil's absorption and increase blood flow to the area, providing a soothing effect.

4. Relax and Unwind: Lie down and relax for at least 30 minutes to allow the oil to work its magic. Use this time to meditate, listen to calming music, or simply breathe deeply.

5. Clean Up: After the time is up, gently wipe away any excess oil with a warm, damp cloth. You can repeat this process several times during your cycle, especially on the first few days when cramps tend to be the most intense.

In addition to topical applications, incorporating castor oil internally can support hormonal balance, potentially reducing the severity of cramps. However, this approach should be done with caution and ideally under the guidance of a healthcare professional, particularly for those unfamiliar with internal use of oils.

Besides topical applications and internal use, lifestyle changes can significantly enhance the effectiveness of castor oil in alleviating menstrual cramps. Regular exercise, for instance, increases blood flow, which can ease cramping. Activities like yoga or gentle stretching can also help relax the pelvic muscles, reducing tension and pain.

Diet plays a crucial role in managing menstrual symptoms as well. Consuming anti-inflammatory foods, such as leafy greens, berries, nuts, and fatty fish, can counteract inflammation and contribute to overall hormonal balance. Staying hydrated is essential too; proper hydration can prevent bloating and discomfort associated with menstrual cycles.

Moreover, consider incorporating herbal teas that complement castor oil's effects. Herbal infusions, such as ginger tea or chamomile tea, have been used traditionally to help with menstrual discomfort. Ginger, for example, is known for its anti-inflammatory properties and can help reduce the severity of cramps. Chamomile, with its calming effects, can promote relaxation and ease tension in the body.

As you explore the benefits of castor oil and these complementary practices, it's important to listen to your body. Every woman's experience with menstrual cramps is unique, and what works for one may not work for another. Keeping a menstrual diary can be a helpful tool; tracking your symptoms, dietary choices, and the efficacy of various remedies can guide you towards what works best for you.

It's equally essential to approach your menstrual health holistically. Stress management techniques, such as mindfulness, meditation, or deep-breathing exercises, can significantly impact how you experience cramps. High stress levels can exacerbate pain perception, making it crucial to incorporate relaxation practices into your routine.

If you find that your cramps are severe or accompanied by other troubling symptoms, consulting with a healthcare provider is vital. While castor oil and natural remedies can be effective for many, they are not a substitute for professional medical advice, especially if you experience debilitating pain or irregularities in your cycle.

By integrating castor oil into your menstrual care routine, you can take control of your discomfort and embrace a more natural approach to health. With its rich history in traditional medicine and a growing body of scientific support, castor oil represents a powerful tool in the journey toward a more comfortable and balanced menstrual experience.

Ultimately, the goal is not just to mask the pain but to understand your body better and empower it to heal naturally. As you embark on this journey with castor oil, remember that self-care is a vital component of women's health—one that can lead to profound improvements not just during menstruation but in your overall well-being. Embrace this opportunity to nurture yourself with nature's gifts, finding solace in the knowledge that effective, natural remedies are at your fingertips.

PMS, or premenstrual syndrome, is a monthly challenge for many women, characterized by a range of physical and emotional symptoms that can disrupt daily life. From mood swings and irritability to bloating, fatigue, and cramps, the toll of PMS can feel overwhelming. While many turn to over-the-counter medications to alleviate these symptoms, castor oil presents a natural, holistic approach that can provide relief without the side effects commonly associated with pharmaceuticals.

One of the key components of castor oil is ricinoleic acid, which has anti-inflammatory properties. This makes castor oil particularly effective for soothing the discomfort often associated with menstrual cramps. The oil can help relax the muscles of the uterus, reducing tension and easing pain. Additionally, its penetration ability allows it to be absorbed into the skin, where it can work directly on the affected areas.

To harness the power of castor oil for PMS relief, consider creating a simple abdominal massage oil. Start with two tablespoons of organic castor oil and add a few drops of essential oils known for their soothing properties, such as lavender or chamomile. These oils not only enhance the aroma but also provide additional calming effects. After combining the oils, warm the mixture slightly (make sure it's comfortable to touch) and gently massage it into your lower abdomen in circular motions. This ritual not only helps alleviate cramps but also promotes relaxation, allowing you to unwind during those challenging days.

Another effective method to utilize castor oil for PMS is through a castor oil pack. This age-old remedy involves saturating a piece of flannel or cotton fabric with castor oil and placing it on the abdomen. Cover the pack with plastic wrap to prevent leakage and apply a heating pad or hot water bottle on top. The heat enhances the oil's absorption, providing deep relief to aching muscles and helping to reduce inflammation. Aim to keep the pack on for about 30 to 60 minutes, allowing the soothing properties of castor oil to work their magic. This practice can be particularly beneficial when done in the evening, as it promotes relaxation and prepares your body for a restful night's sleep.

In addition to topical applications, incorporating castor oil into your diet can also support hormonal balance, which is crucial for alleviating PMS symptoms. Consider adding a teaspoon of cold-pressed castor oil to smoothies or salad dressings. While it has a distinct flavor, when blended with other ingredients, it can provide a nutrient-rich boost. Just be mindful of the quantity, as castor oil can have a laxative effect in larger doses.

Another area where castor oil shines is its ability to support liver health. The liver plays a vital role in hormone regulation, and a healthy liver can lead to more stable hormone levels. By supporting liver function, castor oil may help mitigate some of the hormonal fluctuations that contribute to PMS symptoms. To promote liver health, you can create a detox drink by mixing a teaspoon of castor oil with lemon juice and warm water. This concoction can stimulate liver function and improve digestion, further aiding in your overall well-being.

Hydration is crucial during PMS. Dehydration can exacerbate bloating and fatigue, making symptoms feel even more intense. To help counteract this, consider infusing water with slices of lemon, cucumber, or mint, and drink it throughout the day. While castor oil won't directly hydrate you, maintaining proper fluid intake will support your body's natural detoxification processes, making it easier to manage PMS symptoms.

Dietary choices also play a significant role in managing PMS. Incorporating foods rich in omega-3 fatty acids, such as flaxseeds, walnuts, and fatty fish can help reduce inflammation and mitigate cramps. Magnesium-rich foods like leafy greens, bananas, and dark chocolate can also help alleviate mood swings and irritability. Pairing these dietary strategies with castor oil's benefits can create a comprehensive approach to managing PMS.

Finally, don't underestimate the importance of self-care during your menstrual cycle. Taking time to care for yourself can significantly impact how you feel. Whether it's indulging in a warm bath, practicing yoga, or meditating, these activities can help reduce stress and promote emotional well-being. During these moments, consider incorporating castor oil massages or packs as part of your self-care routine, enhancing both the physical and emotional aspects of your PMS management.

In summary, castor oil offers a versatile and natural approach to easing PMS symptoms. Its anti-inflammatory properties can alleviate cramps, while its liver-supporting benefits can help regulate hormones. By integrating castor oil into your self-care rituals, both topically and internally, you can create a holistic strategy that addresses the root causes of PMS. As you explore these remedies, remember that self-compassion is crucial; listening to your body and responding with kindness can make a world of difference in how you navigate your menstrual cycle. Embrace the natural power of castor oil and take control of your health, allowing yourself to enjoy life fully, even during those challenging days.

Chapter 8: Total Body Detox and Gut Health

Supporting digestion is fundamental to maintaining overall health and well-being. The digestive system is intricately connected to many bodily functions, influencing everything from nutrient absorption and energy levels to immune response and even mood. When digestion is compromised, it can lead to a cascade of issues, including bloating, discomfort, constipation, and even chronic conditions. Fortunately, castor oil offers a natural way to support and enhance digestive health.

Castor oil is derived from the seeds of the castor bean plant, scientifically known as Ricinus communis. This oil has been used for centuries not only for its numerous health benefits but also for its unique composition of fatty acids, particularly ricinoleic acid. This potent compound is known for its anti-inflammatory and laxative properties, making castor oil an effective option for promoting digestive health.

One of the most common uses of castor oil in digestive health is its ability to relieve constipation. The ricinoleic acid in castor oil works by stimulating the intestines, promoting peristalsis — the wave-like muscle contractions that move food through the digestive tract. When taken in moderation, castor oil can provide a gentle yet effective laxative effect, helping to ease discomfort and facilitate regular bowel movements.

If you find yourself struggling with occasional constipation, consider a simple castor oil remedy. Mix one tablespoon of castor oil with a glass of warm water or juice. Drinking this mixture on an empty stomach can help stimulate bowel activity. However, it's essential to remember that while castor oil can be a helpful occasional remedy, it should not be relied on as a long-term solution for digestive issues. Chronic constipation may require a more comprehensive approach, including dietary adjustments and increased fiber intake.

In addition to its laxative properties, castor oil can also support gut health by acting as a natural anti-inflammatory agent. Inflammatory conditions of the digestive tract, such as irritable bowel syndrome (IBS) and inflammatory bowel disease (IBD), can benefit from the soothing effects of castor oil. By reducing inflammation, castor oil may help alleviate symptoms such as cramping, bloating, and discomfort.

To harness the anti-inflammatory properties of castor oil, consider incorporating it into your daily routine in a gentle, holistic manner. You might use it as a massage oil to soothe your abdomen, applying a warm compress over the area to enhance its effects. Warmth helps to relax the muscles of the digestive tract, promoting improved blood circulation and further alleviating discomfort.

Another valuable aspect of castor oil is its role in detoxification. The digestive system is responsible for processing and eliminating waste, toxins, and byproducts of metabolism. When the digestive system is sluggish or not functioning optimally, these toxins can accumulate, leading to various health issues. Castor oil can aid in detoxifying the body by promoting liver function and enhancing bile production, which is essential for fat digestion and the elimination of waste.

A simple detoxifying routine can be established by incorporating castor oil into your wellness practices. One effective method is to perform a castor oil pack. To create a castor oil pack, you'll need a piece of flannel or cotton fabric, castor oil, plastic wrap, and a heating pad. Start by soaking the fabric in castor oil, then place it over your abdomen. Cover it with plastic wrap to prevent any oil from leaking, and apply a heating pad over the pack to help the oil penetrate the skin. Relax for 30 to 60 minutes while the pack works its magic. This practice can help promote liver health, improve digestion, and enhance overall detoxification.

In addition to these remedies, consider pairing castor oil with other natural digestive aids to create a more comprehensive approach to gut health. Probiotic-rich foods, such as yogurt, kefir, and fermented vegetables, can help replenish beneficial gut bacteria, supporting digestion. Additionally, incorporating digestive enzymes and fiber-rich foods such as fruits, vegetables, and whole grains can further enhance digestive function.

Staying hydrated is equally important for optimal digestion. Water supports every aspect of your digestive process, from breaking down food to transporting nutrients. Aim to drink at least eight glasses of water a day, and consider starting your morning with a glass of warm water and lemon to kickstart your digestive system.

As you work to support your digestion naturally, it's essential to be mindful of your body's signals. Pay attention to how different foods affect your digestive health and make adjustments as necessary. Keeping a food diary can be a helpful way to track patterns, allowing you to identify triggers and better understand your body's unique needs.

While castor oil can be a powerful ally in supporting digestion, it's crucial to approach it with respect and care. Always consult with a healthcare professional before starting any new health regimen, especially if you have underlying health conditions or are taking medications. They can help guide you in using castor oil safely and effectively.

In conclusion, embracing castor oil as part of your digestive health toolkit can lead to significant improvements in your overall wellness. From easing constipation to reducing inflammation and supporting detoxification, this versatile oil offers a myriad of benefits for your digestive system. By incorporating castor oil into your routine alongside a balanced diet, hydration, and mindful practices, you can pave the way for a happier, healthier gut. Remember, health is a journey, and every small step you take brings you closer to achieving optimal well-being.

The liver is one of the body's most vital organs, acting as a natural filter that cleanses the bloodstream and processes nutrients from the food we consume. It plays an essential role in detoxification, metabolizing drugs and alcohol, and producing bile for digestion. Given its numerous functions, maintaining liver health is crucial for overall well-being. When the liver becomes overloaded with toxins—whether from environmental pollutants, unhealthy foods, or excessive alcohol consumption—it can lead to a host of health issues. This is where castor oil can be a powerful ally in restoring liver balance and supporting your body’s natural detoxification processes.

One of the primary ways castor oil contributes to liver health is through its unique composition of ricinoleic acid. This fatty acid possesses anti-inflammatory properties that can help reduce inflammation in the liver. Inflammation is often a precursor to more serious liver conditions, including fatty liver disease and cirrhosis. By incorporating castor oil into your routine, you can promote a healthier liver environment, reducing the risk of such conditions while enhancing your body’s ability to detoxify.

The detoxifying effects of castor oil extend beyond the liver. When absorbed through the skin, it can stimulate lymphatic flow, which is essential for removing toxins from the body. The lymphatic system works in tandem with the liver, as it helps transport waste products to the liver for processing. By using castor oil in a topical application, you can indirectly support liver function and enhance your body's detoxification pathways.

For those interested in a more direct approach to liver cleansing, castor oil packs are an excellent option. A castor oil pack involves saturating a piece of cloth with castor oil, placing it over the liver area, and covering it with plastic wrap to prevent messiness. This application can be secured with a heating pad or hot water bottle to enhance absorption. The warmth increases blood circulation, helping the oil penetrate deeper into the tissues and providing relief from any discomfort or tension in the area. Regular use of castor oil packs can promote liver detoxification, enhance circulation, and support overall liver function.

When creating a castor oil pack, it's important to choose high-quality, cold-pressed castor oil. This ensures that you're getting the oil in its purest form, maximizing its beneficial properties. To prepare your pack, follow these simple steps:

1. **Gather Your Materials**: You'll need a clean, soft cotton cloth (preferably flannel), plastic wrap, a heating pad or hot water bottle, and, of course, castor oil.

2. **Saturate the Cloth**: Pour a generous amount of castor oil onto the cloth until it's thoroughly saturated but not dripping.

3. **Apply the Pack**: Lie down in a comfortable position and place the saturated cloth over your liver, which is located on your right side, just below the rib cage.

4. **Cover with Plastic**: Place plastic wrap over the cloth to keep it in place and prevent any oil from seeping onto your bedding.

5. **Add Heat**: Place your heating pad or hot water bottle over the pack. The heat will help the oil penetrate the skin and enhance its detoxifying effects.

6. **Relax**: Allow the pack to sit for 30 to 60 minutes. Use this time to relax—read a book, meditate, or simply enjoy some quiet time.

7. **Clean Up**: After your session, clean the area with a mild soap and water to remove any residual oil.

In addition to topical applications, integrating castor oil into your diet can also support liver health. Castor oil is known for its laxative properties, which can stimulate bowel movements and help eliminate waste from the digestive system. However, it should be used in moderation. A common approach is to take one teaspoon of castor oil mixed with a glass of juice or water once a week to aid digestion and promote regularity. Always consult with a healthcare professional before starting any new supplement regimen, especially if you have any pre-existing health conditions.

Hydration is another critical factor in maintaining liver health. Drinking plenty of water helps dilute toxins in the bloodstream, allowing the liver to process them more efficiently. Consider adding lemon juice to your water, as the citric acid can enhance the liver's detoxification processes. The combination of hydration and the detoxifying properties of castor oil creates a powerful synergy that can help restore balance to your liver and promote overall health.

Incorporating a healthy, balanced diet rich in whole foods is equally important for liver health. Foods such as leafy greens, cruciferous vegetables, berries, and nuts provide essential nutrients that support liver function. Antioxidants found in these foods can help neutralize harmful free radicals, reducing oxidative stress on the liver. Additionally, avoiding processed foods, excessive sugar, and unhealthy fats can significantly reduce the burden on your liver, allowing it to function optimally.

As you embark on your journey towards improved liver health, remember that consistency is key. Regular use of castor oil, whether through topical applications, dietary incorporation, or detoxifying packs, can yield significant benefits over time. It's also essential to listen to your body; if you experience any discomfort or adverse reactions, discontinue use and consult with a healthcare professional.

In summary, castor oil offers a versatile and natural approach to cleansing and restoring liver balance. By embracing this ancient remedy, you can support your body's detoxification processes, reduce inflammation, and promote overall wellness. Whether through topical applications, dietary integration, or holistic practices, castor oil can be an invaluable addition to your health routine. As you nurture your liver health, you'll likely notice improvements in your overall energy levels, digestion, and vitality—empowering you to lead a healthier, more vibrant life.

Detoxification is an essential process that our bodies undergo naturally, but sometimes, they need a little help to function optimally. In a world filled with toxins—from environmental pollutants to processed foods—supporting our body's natural detox mechanisms can lead to significant improvements in health, energy levels, and overall well-being. Natural detox methods often harness the power of whole foods, herbs, and simple lifestyle changes, making them not only effective but also easy to incorporate into daily routines.

To begin, let's consider the importance of staying hydrated. Water is vital for all bodily functions, including detoxification. It aids in flushing out toxins through urine and sweat, while also helping to transport nutrients and oxygen to cells. Aim for at least eight glasses of water a day, and consider adding fresh lemon juice to your water for an extra detox boost. Lemon aids liver function, enhances digestion, and provides a rich source of vitamin C, which is crucial for neutralizing free radicals.

In addition to hydration, consider the role of dietary choices in detoxification. A diet rich in fruits, vegetables, whole grains, and lean proteins provides the nutrients your body needs to effectively eliminate toxins. Cruciferous vegetables like broccoli, cauliflower, and kale are known for their powerful detoxifying properties. They contain compounds that support liver health—our primary detoxifying organ—by promoting the production of enzymes needed for detoxification. Incorporating garlic, onions, and leeks into your meals can further enhance liver function due to their sulfur-containing compounds, which help to detoxify heavy metals and other harmful substances.

Fiber is another crucial component in a detox diet. It aids in digestion and helps to move waste through the digestive tract, reducing the risk of constipation and promoting regular bowel movements. Foods high in fiber include legumes, whole grains, nuts, seeds, fruits, and vegetables. Consider starting your day with a fiber-rich breakfast of oatmeal topped with berries and seeds or a smoothie loaded with spinach, banana, and chia seeds. This not only supports detoxification but also keeps you feeling full and energized throughout the day.

Herbal teas can also play a significant role in natural detox methods. Certain herbs possess properties that stimulate liver function, improve digestion, and support kidney health. Dandelion root tea is particularly beneficial; it acts as a diuretic, promoting urine production and helping to eliminate excess water and toxins. Green tea, rich in antioxidants known as catechins, enhances liver function and boosts metabolism. Consider replacing your afternoon coffee with a cup of herbal tea to reap these detox benefits.

Another excellent natural detox method is through the practice of intermittent fasting. This approach allows your body to enter a state of autophagy, during which it cleanses and repairs itself by breaking down and eliminating damaged cells and proteins. Intermittent fasting can take various forms, such as the 16/8 method (fasting for 16 hours and eating within an 8-hour window) or the 5:2 method (eating normally for five days and significantly reducing calorie intake for two non-consecutive days). This practice not only supports detoxification but can also lead to improved mental clarity and energy levels.

Incorporating physical activity into your routine is another powerful detox method. Exercise promotes circulation, helps to eliminate toxins through sweat, and enhances overall metabolic function. Whether it's a brisk walk, a yoga session, or a high-intensity workout, find an activity you enjoy and make it a regular part of your week. Aim for at least 150 minutes of moderate-intensity exercise per week, and don't forget to incorporate deep breathing techniques. Deep breathing can help to oxygenate your blood and release built-up tension, allowing for a more effective detox process on a cellular level.

Sleep is often an overlooked aspect of detoxification. Quality sleep is essential for the body to repair itself and eliminate toxins accumulated throughout the day. During sleep, the brain undergoes a cleansing process known as the glymphatic system, which removes waste products. Aim for 7-9 hours of quality sleep each night. Establishing a calming bedtime routine—such as dimming the lights, avoiding screens, and engaging in relaxation techniques like meditation or gentle stretching—can significantly improve your sleep quality.

Finally, consider incorporating castor oil into your detox routine. Known for its powerful detoxifying properties, castor oil can be used in various ways to support liver health and enhance digestion. A popular method is the castor oil pack, where a cloth soaked in warm castor oil is placed over the abdomen. This can help to stimulate circulation and promote lymphatic drainage, making it an excellent addition to your detox practices. For best results, use the pack for 30-60 minutes a few times a week, and always remember to cover your skin with a towel to avoid any mess.

Incorporating these natural detox methods into your life doesn't have to be overwhelming. Start with small changes, such as drinking more water, adding a few extra servings of fruits and vegetables to your meals, or trying a new herbal tea. Over time, these adjustments will become a part of your routine, leading to a healthier, more vibrant you. Remember, detoxification is not a one-time event but a continuous process that can be supported through mindful choices and a holistic approach to health. By embracing these natural methods, you empower your body to function at its best, allowing you to thrive in every aspect of your life.

Chapter 9: Crafting with Castor Oil

Homemade soaps crafted with castor oil bring a luxurious touch to your daily hygiene routine, transforming what is often a mundane task into a delightful experience. The benefits of castor oil extend beyond its health and beauty applications; it also plays an essential role in creating soaps that nourish, moisturize, and rejuvenate the skin.

Castor oil, derived from the seeds of the Ricinus communis plant, is rich in ricinoleic acid, a fatty acid known for its anti-inflammatory, antimicrobial, and skin-conditioning properties. This makes it an excellent ingredient for soap-making, offering a myriad of benefits that enhance the quality of the final product.

One of the standout features of castor oil in homemade soap is its ability to create a rich, creamy lather. Unlike some oils that may produce a more bubbly, airy foam, castor oil generates a dense, luxurious lather that feels indulgent on the skin. This is particularly beneficial for those with dry or sensitive skin, as it provides a moisturizing effect that keeps the skin hydrated even after washing. The soap glides smoothly over the skin, allowing for an enjoyable bathing experience that leaves you feeling refreshed rather than stripped of natural oils.

When making soap, it's essential to balance the properties of different oils to achieve the desired outcome. Castor oil is often used in combination with other oils such as olive, coconut, and palm oils. Each oil contributes unique qualities: olive oil offers conditioning and antioxidant benefits; coconut oil produces a bubbly lather; and palm oil provides hardness and stability to the soap. By incorporating castor oil into your recipes, you can create a well-rounded bar that showcases the best features of each ingredient.

Beyond its lathering capabilities, castor oil is known for its skin-soothing properties. It is particularly effective at alleviating dryness and irritation, making it an ideal choice for those with conditions such as eczema or psoriasis. The anti-inflammatory properties of ricinoleic acid can help calm inflamed skin, providing relief from discomfort while promoting healing. When you use castor oil soap, you're not just cleaning your skin; you're also treating it to a nourishing experience that helps maintain its natural barrier.

One of the most significant advantages of making your own soap is the ability to control the ingredients. Many commercial soaps contain synthetic additives, fragrances, and preservatives that can irritate the skin or cause allergic reactions. By using pure, organic castor oil and other natural ingredients, you can create a product that is free from harmful chemicals, ensuring a gentle touch for even the most sensitive skin types.

To start crafting your own castor oil soap, you'll need a few basic supplies: a soap-making kit, which typically includes a scale, thermometer, stick blender, and molds; ingredients like oils, lye, and any optional additives such as essential oils, herbs, or natural colorants; and a workspace that is well-ventilated and protected. Safety is paramount when using lye, as it is corrosive and can cause burns. Always wear gloves and goggles, and follow all safety guidelines when handling this chemical.

There are two primary methods for making soap: cold process and hot process. The cold process method allows you to create a soap that retains the beneficial properties of the oils, including castor oil. In this method, lye is mixed with water to create a lye solution, which is then combined with the oils. The mixture is blended until it reaches "trace," a stage where it thickens and leaves a trail on the surface when drizzled. Once trace is achieved, you can add any desired fragrances or colorants before pouring the mixture into molds to set.

If you choose the hot process method, the soap undergoes a cooking process that accelerates saponification—the chemical reaction that turns oils and lye into soap. This method allows you to use your soap sooner, as it doesn't require as long to cure. However, it may not yield the same creamy lather as cold process soap.

When crafting your soap, consider adding additional nourishing ingredients to enhance the properties of castor oil. Essential oils, such as lavender or tea tree oil, not only provide pleasant fragrances but also impart additional benefits, such as antibacterial properties or calming effects. You can also experiment with natural exfoliants like oatmeal, coffee grounds, or dried herbs to create a textured soap that gently exfoliates the skin.

As you begin your soap-making journey, don't be afraid to experiment with different combinations and techniques. Keep a journal to document your recipes, observations, and results. This will not only help you refine your skills but also allow you to create personalized soaps that cater to your specific preferences and skin needs.

Once your soap is ready, you can enjoy the many benefits it offers. Use it daily to cleanse your skin while treating it to the nourishing effects of castor oil. The result will be a bar of soap that not only smells divine but also leaves your skin feeling soft, hydrated, and radiant.

Moreover, homemade castor oil soap makes for thoughtful gifts. Wrapping your creations in beautiful packaging or labeling them with their unique benefits adds a personal touch that friends and family will appreciate. Share your knowledge and passion for natural skincare with loved ones, empowering them to embrace a healthier lifestyle.

In conclusion, crafting homemade soaps with castor oil is not just a fun and creative endeavor; it is also an opportunity to enhance your skin health and wellness naturally. By utilizing the remarkable properties of castor oil, you can create a product that not only cleans but also nourishes and rejuvenates. So roll up your sleeves, gather your ingredients, and immerse yourself in the art of soap-making. Your skin will thank you!

Creating candles with castor oil is an exciting and fulfilling way to harness the benefits of this versatile oil while indulging in a creative hobby. Not only do homemade candles provide a warm, inviting ambiance, but they also allow you to infuse your space with natural scents and therapeutic properties. Castor oil, known for its moisturizing and soothing qualities, can be a wonderful addition to your candle-making repertoire. Let's explore how to make your own castor oil candles, including the benefits, materials needed, and step-by-step instructions.

To begin, let's discuss why castor oil is an excellent choice for candle-making. Traditionally, candles are made from waxes like paraffin, beeswax, or soy, which can sometimes lack the nourishing properties that castor oil offers. When incorporated into your candles, castor oil not only helps moisturize the skin but also enhances the scent throw, allowing fragrances to disperse more effectively throughout your space. Furthermore, castor oil burns cleanly, resulting in a longer-lasting candle with a gentle, soft glow.

Before you start crafting your castor oil candles, you'll need to gather your materials. The basic supplies include:

1. **Wax**: You can choose from a variety of waxes, including soy wax, beeswax, or a paraffin blend. Soy wax is particularly popular for its clean burn and ease of use.

2. **Castor Oil**: Look for high-quality, cold-pressed castor oil to ensure that you're using the best possible ingredient.

3. **Wicks**: Choose cotton or wooden wicks, depending on your preference. Make sure the wick size is appropriate for the diameter of your candle.

4. **Fragrance Oils or Essential Oils**: This is where you can get creative! You can use essential oils like lavender, eucalyptus, or citrus for a natural scent or opt for synthetic fragrance oils that offer a wider variety of fragrances.

5. **Containers or Molds**: Glass jars, metal tins, or silicone molds work well for pouring your candles. Make sure they are heat-resistant and can accommodate the wax.

6. **Double Boiler**: This is essential for melting your wax safely without burning it. If you don't have a double boiler, you can create one by placing a heat-safe bowl over a pot of simmering water.

7. **Thermometer**: Keeping track of the temperature is crucial for the proper blending of wax and oil.

Once you have your materials ready, it's time to dive into the candle-making process. Follow these simple steps to create your own castor oil candles:

Step 1: Measure Your Wax Start by determining how much wax you will need based on the size of your container. A good rule of thumb is to use one ounce of wax for every ounce of the container's volume. For instance, if your jar holds 8 ounces, you'll need 8 ounces of wax.

Step 2: Melt the Wax Using your double boiler, heat the wax gently until it is fully melted. Monitor the temperature with your thermometer; it should reach around 170–180°F (77–82°C). Be careful not to overheat it, as this can affect the scent throw and the burning quality of the candle.

Step 3: Add Castor Oil Once your wax is melted, it's time to incorporate the castor oil. For a well-balanced candle, use about 10-15% castor oil in relation to the total weight of the wax. For example, if you are using 8 ounces of wax, add 0.8 to 1.2 ounces of castor oil. Stir well to ensure the oil is evenly distributed throughout the wax.

Step 4: Add Fragrance If you're adding fragrance oils or essential oils, do so after mixing in the castor oil. The ideal amount of fragrance is typically 6-10% of the total weight of the wax. For an 8-ounce batch, this would mean adding approximately 0.5 to 0.8 ounces of fragrance. Stir thoroughly for a couple of minutes, allowing the fragrance to bind well with the wax blend.

Step 5: Prepare Your Wick While your wax is cooling slightly, prepare your wick. If you're using a container, secure the wick to the bottom using a dab of melted wax or a wick sticker. Make sure the wick stands upright and is centered in the container.

Step 6: Pour the Wax Once the wax temperature has dropped to around 150-160°F (65-71°C), carefully pour it into your prepared container. Make sure to pour slowly and steadily to avoid air bubbles. Fill your container, leaving a bit of space at the top.

Step 7: Secure the Wick To keep the wick centered while the candle sets, you can use a wick holder or simply lay a chopstick or pencil across the top of the container, securing the wick in place.

Step 8: Allow to Cool Let your candle cool completely, which may take several hours. Avoid moving the candle during this time, as it can create uneven surfaces or cracks.

Step 9: Trim the Wick Once your candle has fully cooled and solidified, trim the wick to about ¼ inch above the wax surface. This will help prevent excessive soot and ensure a clean burn.

Step 10: Cure Your Candle For the best scent throw and burn quality, allow your candle to cure for at least a few days before lighting it. This waiting period helps the fragrance fully develop and bind with the wax.

Now that you have your castor oil candle, it's time to enjoy the fruits of your labor! Light it up and revel in the soothing aroma, knowing that you've created something beautiful and beneficial for your environment.

Creating candles with castor oil not only enhances your home but also serves as a wonderful way to practice self-care. Whether you choose to make them for yourself or as heartfelt gifts for loved ones, these candles will surely brighten any space and provide a touch of natural wellness. So gather your supplies, unleash your creativity, and enjoy the therapeutic benefits of candle-making with castor oil!

Crafting with castor oil opens up a world of possibilities, allowing you to create a variety of natural products that are not only effective but also free from harmful chemicals. In this section, we will explore 50 DIY recipes for home use, showcasing the versatility of castor oil in everything from skin care to household items. These recipes will help you harness the benefits of castor oil while enjoying the satisfaction of making your own products.

Starting with skin care, castor oil is a powerful ingredient that can be incorporated into several recipes for a nourishing and rejuvenating experience. One delightful option is a castor oil face mask, perfect for moisturizing and detoxifying the skin. Combine two tablespoons of castor oil with one tablespoon of honey and one tablespoon of yogurt. Apply this mixture to your face, leave it on for 15-20 minutes, then rinse off with warm water. Your skin will feel soft, hydrated, and glowing.

For those dealing with acne or blemishes, a castor oil spot treatment can be a game-changer. Mix equal parts castor oil and tea tree oil, then apply directly to problem areas with a cotton swab. Tea tree oil's antibacterial properties, combined with castor oil's moisturizing benefits, work wonders in reducing inflammation and promoting healthier skin.

Another must-try is a luxurious body scrub that exfoliates while nourishing the skin. Combine half a cup of brown sugar, half a cup of castor oil, and a few drops of your favorite essential oil, such as lavender or eucalyptus. Mix well and use this scrub in the shower to slough off dead skin cells and leave your skin silky smooth.

Moving on to hair care, castor oil is renowned for its ability to promote hair growth and overall scalp health. A simple castor oil hair mask can be made by mixing two tablespoons of castor oil with one tablespoon of coconut oil and a few drops of rosemary essential oil. Apply this mixture to your hair and scalp, leave it on for at least 30 minutes, then wash it out with your regular shampoo. Regular use can lead to thicker, healthier hair.

For a nourishing beard oil, blend one tablespoon of castor oil with two tablespoons of argan oil and a few drops of cedarwood essential oil. This concoction not only nourishes the hair but also promotes growth and adds a pleasant scent.

In addition to beauty products, castor oil can also be used to create household items. For instance, making your own natural furniture polish is incredibly simple. Combine one cup of castor oil with half a cup of vinegar and a few drops of lemon essential oil. This mixture will not only clean your wooden furniture but also leave it shining and smelling fresh.

You can also create a natural insect repellent using castor oil. Combine one cup of water, two tablespoons of castor oil, and a few drops of peppermint essential oil in a spray bottle. Shake well before each use and spray around doorways and windows to deter pests while keeping your home smelling delightful.

For those interested in personal care, consider crafting your own natural deodorant. Mix two tablespoons of castor oil with three tablespoons of baking soda, one tablespoon of cornstarch, and a few drops of your favorite essential oil. Store this mixture in a small jar and apply it as needed for a fresh, chemical-free alternative to commercial deodorants.

If you're looking to create a soothing massage oil, combine three tablespoons of castor oil with two tablespoons of sweet almond oil and a few drops of lavender essential oil. This blend is perfect for easing muscle tension and promoting relaxation after a long day.

Now, let's explore some creative uses for castor oil beyond personal care. You can make homemade candles that are not only beautiful but also eco-friendly. Melt one cup of beeswax and one cup of castor oil together over low heat. Once melted, add a few drops of your favorite essential oil for fragrance. Pour the mixture into a mold with a wick and allow it to cool completely. Enjoy the warm glow and soothing scent of your homemade candle.

Another interesting recipe is for homemade soap. Combine 16 ounces of coconut oil, 16 ounces of olive oil, and 8 ounces of castor oil in a heat-safe container. In a separate container, mix 12 ounces of lye with 32 ounces of distilled water (always add lye to water, never the other way around). Once both mixtures have cooled, slowly combine them, stirring until trace is achieved. Pour the mixture into a mold and allow it to cure for several weeks before using. This soap will be gentle on the skin and provide a rich lather.

For a fun, family-friendly project, consider making castor oil-infused bath bombs. Mix one cup of baking soda, half a cup of citric acid, half a cup of Epsom salt, and half a cup of castor oil in a bowl. Add a few drops of essential oil for fragrance and mix until the consistency resembles damp sand. Pack the mixture tightly into molds and let them dry for 24 hours. Enjoy these fizzy delights in your bath for a relaxing experience.

For cleaning purposes, you can create a natural all-purpose cleaner using castor oil. Mix one cup of water, one cup of white vinegar, and a tablespoon of castor oil in a spray bottle. This cleaner is effective for various surfaces around the house and eliminates the need for harsh chemicals.

Lastly, if you have pets, castor oil can be beneficial for their coat as well. Combine two tablespoons of castor oil with one tablespoon of olive oil and massage it into your pet's coat. This mixture can help reduce shedding and promote a shiny, healthy appearance.

These 50 DIY recipes demonstrate the incredible versatility of castor oil, making it an essential ingredient for anyone looking to embrace natural living. By incorporating these creations into your routine, you can enjoy the myriad benefits of castor oil while reducing reliance on commercial products. Whether for personal care, home cleaning, or crafting, castor oil provides a simple yet effective solution to enhance your lifestyle. Embrace the art of crafting with castor oil and let your creativity flourish!

Chapter 10: Incorporating Castor Oil into Daily Routine

Establishing a healthy routine that incorporates castor oil can transform not only your beauty regimen but also your overall wellness. The key to successfully integrating this powerful oil into your daily life lies in consistency, mindfulness, and creativity. By making castor oil a staple in your self-care rituals, you'll harness its myriad benefits while fostering a deeper connection to your own health and beauty journey.

To begin, it's essential to assess your current lifestyle and identify areas where castor oil can seamlessly fit in. Whether you are seeking to rejuvenate your skin, stimulate hair growth, or relieve minor aches and pains, having a clear understanding of your goals will guide your routine. Take a moment to reflect on what you hope to achieve with castor oil. Are you struggling with dry skin? Do you want thicker eyebrows or fuller lashes? Perhaps you're dealing with digestive issues or joint discomfort. Whatever your focus, establishing specific goals will give you a sense of direction and purpose as you embark on this journey.

Once you've established your objectives, the next step is to create a structured routine that incorporates castor oil in a way that feels natural and enjoyable. Here are some strategies to help you design a daily regimen that aligns with your goals:

1. **Morning Rituals**: Start your day with intention. Incorporate castor oil into your morning skincare routine by using it as a moisturizer. A few drops can be warmed in your hands and gently massaged into your face. This not only hydrates your skin but also promotes circulation, giving you a healthy glow to start

the day. If you're focused on hair health, consider applying castor oil to your scalp and hair ends as a pre-shampoo treatment. This will nourish your hair and prepare it for cleansing.

2. **Midday Boost**: As the day progresses, you may find moments where you can take a breather. Consider carrying a small bottle of castor oil with you for on-the-go skincare. If your skin feels dry or irritated, a quick application can provide instant relief. For those looking to enhance their brows or lashes, applying a tiny amount of castor oil with a clean mascara wand can be a simple yet effective lunchtime ritual. This not only nourishes your hair follicles but also allows you to indulge in a few moments of self-care.

3. **Evening Unwind**: Establishing a nighttime routine is crucial for promoting relaxation and preparing your body for restful sleep. After a long day, set aside time for a calming bath or shower. You can create a luxurious experience by adding castor oil to your bathwater, which will help hydrate your skin while you soak. Additionally, consider using castor oil as a massage oil to unwind tense muscles. A gentle massage on sore joints or tight areas can work wonders in relieving discomfort and promoting relaxation.

4. **Weekly Treatments**: To maximize the benefits of castor oil, incorporate it into your routine on a weekly basis. Designate a specific day for deep treatments. For example, on Sundays, you might choose to apply a castor oil hair mask, allowing it to penetrate your hair and scalp for several hours or overnight for intense nourishment. Similarly, you could reserve time for a facial with castor oil as the star ingredient, mixing it with other natural components like honey or essential oils for added benefits.

5. **Mindful Journaling**: As you establish this routine, consider keeping a wellness journal to track your experiences and results. Document how your skin and hair respond to the weekly treatments, any changes in your health, and how you feel overall. Journaling helps cultivate mindfulness, making you more aware of your body's responses and reinforcing the positive habits you're creating. Reflecting on your journey will not only motivate you to continue but also allow you to make adjustments as needed.

6. **Be Flexible**: Incorporating a new element into your routine should never feel like a chore. It's essential to remain flexible and adapt your practices as needed. If you discover that certain applications aren't working for you or if your schedule changes, don't hesitate to modify your routine. The beauty of using castor oil lies in its versatility; you can use it in numerous ways to suit your lifestyle. Experiment with different methods of application, ratios, and combinations with other natural ingredients to find what resonates best with you.

7. **Community and Support**: Finally, consider reaching out to communities that share your interests in natural remedies and holistic health. Engaging with others who are also incorporating castor oil into their routines can provide inspiration, motivation, and a sense of camaraderie. Share your successes and challenges, exchange ideas for new recipes, and learn from their experiences. This shared journey can enhance your commitment to your routine and create an uplifting environment for your self-care practices.

As you weave castor oil into the fabric of your daily life, remember that establishing a healthy routine is a journey, not a destination. Embrace the process and celebrate your progress, no matter how small. The benefits you begin to experience—glowing skin, stronger hair, pain relief, and improved overall wellness—will be well worth the effort. With consistent use of castor oil and a mindful approach to self-care, you'll not only achieve your health and beauty goals but also cultivate a deeper appreciation for your body and its natural abilities. Now, take a deep breath, embrace the journey ahead, and allow the golden oil to transform your life in ways you've always dreamed possible.

Incorporating castor oil into your daily routine can be a transformative experience, but the key to reaping its full benefits lies in consistency. Just like any health regimen, the results you seek will not manifest overnight. However, with a few practical strategies, you can seamlessly integrate castor oil into your everyday life, ensuring that it becomes an essential part of your wellness journey. Here are some thoughtful tips to help you maintain a consistent usage of this remarkable oil.

First and foremost, establish a designated time for your castor oil rituals. Whether it's in the morning, during your evening self-care routine, or at a time that best fits your lifestyle, creating a specific time slot can help you remember to use it regularly. For many, incorporating castor oil into their skincare regimen before bed works wonders. Not only does this allow the oil to work overnight, but it also creates a calming ritual that signals your body it's time to wind down. Consider creating a small self-care corner in your bathroom or bedroom, complete with your castor oil and any other skincare products you enjoy. Having a dedicated space can serve as a visual reminder and make the process feel more intentional.

Another effective strategy is to pair your castor oil usage with activities you already do. For example, if you have a morning routine that includes skincare, consider adding a few drops of castor oil to your moisturizer or using it alone as a hydrating treatment. If you enjoy a weekly hair mask, make it a point to include castor oil as a key ingredient in your treatment. By linking castor oil with existing habits, you're more likely to remember to use it, and you'll also find that it enhances your overall self-care experience.

Keeping a journal can also be incredibly beneficial for tracking your progress and celebrating your milestones. Document how your skin, hair, or overall well-being changes over time as you incorporate castor oil into your routine. Not only will this help you stay motivated, but it can also serve as a powerful reminder of the positive effects you are experiencing. You might even find that documenting your journey allows you to discover new ways to use castor oil that you hadn't considered before.

Moreover, consider investing in a quality castor oil product that you genuinely enjoy using. The sensory experience of the oil—its texture, scent, and how it feels on your skin or hair—can play a significant role in your commitment to using it consistently. Look for organic, cold-pressed castor oil to ensure you're using a pure product. If you enjoy the way it feels and smells, you'll be far more likely to reach for it regularly.

Creating a habit tracker can also be a handy tool to ensure you're using castor oil consistently. You can create a simple chart on paper or use an app on your smartphone to log your usage. Set a goal for how often you want to use castor oil each week and check off each time you do. Seeing your progress visually can reinforce your commitment and motivate you to keep going.

It's also essential to educate yourself about the various ways castor oil can be used. The versatility of this oil is one of its most appealing features. From skincare and haircare to alleviating pain or enhancing digestion, there are numerous applications for castor oil. The more you learn about its uses, the easier it will be to incorporate it into your daily life. For instance, if you discover that castor oil can help with joint pain, you might find it beneficial to apply it regularly after a workout or during your evening relaxation routine.

In addition to its skincare and haircare benefits, consider integrating castor oil into your diet. Many people enjoy taking castor oil internally for its laxative properties or to support gut health. If you choose this route, be sure to consult with a healthcare professional to determine the best approach for your individual needs. Once you understand how castor oil can support your overall wellness, you may find yourself more motivated to use it consistently.

Another way to enhance your commitment to using castor oil is to involve your family and friends. Share your journey and educate those close to you about the benefits of this remarkable oil. You might even host a DIY night where you create castor oil beauty treatments together. When you engage others in your wellness journey, it not only reinforces your own commitment but also fosters a supportive environment where everyone can learn and grow.

Finally, remember to be patient with yourself. Consistency does not mean perfection. Life can be unpredictable, and there may be times when you forget to use castor oil or find it challenging to fit it into your schedule. Acknowledge these moments without guilt, and simply return to your routine when you can. The goal is progress, not perfection. Celebrate the small victories, whether it's noticing healthier hair, smoother skin, or reduced pain. Each positive change is a testament to your commitment to your health and well-being.

As you embark on your journey with castor oil, these strategies will help you maintain consistency and integrate this powerful oil into your daily routine seamlessly. By making castor oil a regular part of your self-care, you'll unlock its full potential and discover the myriad ways it can enhance your beauty and overall health. Embrace the journey and let the golden oil work its magic!

Tracking your progress and results when incorporating castor oil into your daily routine is an essential part of your wellness journey. It not only helps you stay motivated but also allows you to understand how your body responds to this potent natural remedy. With its myriad benefits, from skin rejuvenation to hair transformation and pain relief, being mindful of your progress can enhance your experience and outcomes significantly.

To start tracking your progress, it's helpful to establish a baseline. This means taking some time to assess your current state before you begin using castor oil. For your skin, take clear photographs in natural light to document your complexion, focusing on areas of concern such as acne, wrinkles, or dryness. Note the texture, tone, and any specific issues you want to address. For your hair, take photos of your scalp and strands, paying attention to areas that may be thinning or lacking shine. If you're using castor oil for pain relief, document your pain levels on a scale of one to ten, and note how often you experience discomfort.

Once you have your baseline, create a dedicated journal, either physical or digital, to log your daily or weekly experiences with castor oil. This journal can serve multiple purposes: it's a space for you to record treatments, the frequency of application, and any changes you notice in your skin, hair, or overall well-being.

Consider including the recipes you're trying, how they feel during application, and any immediate effects you observe.

When writing in your journal, it's beneficial to adopt a holistic approach. Instead of only focusing on physical changes, also note emotional and psychological shifts. For instance, do you feel more confident with clearer skin? Are you experiencing less anxiety regarding your hair thinning? Recognizing these emotional benefits can be just as motivating as physical transformations, reinforcing your commitment to incorporating castor oil into your routine.

It's also essential to be patient and realistic about your expectations. Natural remedies like castor oil often take time to show visible results, particularly when it comes to skin and hair health. While some individuals might notice improvements within a week, others could take several weeks or even months to experience significant changes. Documenting these fluctuations can help you maintain a balanced perspective and avoid the disappointment that sometimes accompanies slower progress.

To further enhance your tracking, consider setting specific, measurable goals related to your use of castor oil. For example, you might aim to use a particular treatment three times a week for a month and then assess the results. Or, you could plan to take weekly photographs of your hair or skin for a designated period, allowing you to visually track your progress over time. Setting clear goals not only helps you stay organized but also gives you something concrete to work toward.

Regularly reviewing your journal can provide insights into patterns and results that might not be immediately apparent. For instance, you may notice that certain recipes work better for your skin type or that specific application techniques yield better results. This reflective practice can empower you to adapt your approach as you continue your journey with castor oil.

As you track your progress, it's also worth considering the role of your overall lifestyle in conjunction with the benefits of castor oil. Are you also drinking enough water, eating a balanced diet, or engaging in regular exercise? These factors can significantly influence your results, and being mindful of them can help you identify what works best for your body. If you notice a plateau or a decline in results, it may be an opportunity to reassess other aspects of your health and wellness routine.

Engaging with an online community or support group can further enrich your experience. Sharing your journey with others who are also exploring the benefits of castor oil can provide encouragement, inspiration, and accountability. You may find that others have faced similar challenges or have discovered unique approaches that could enhance your own experience. Plus, the camaraderie and shared successes can be incredibly motivating.

Another valuable method of tracking results is to conduct periodic self-assessments. Set aside time every month or so to evaluate your progress in a more structured manner. You can revisit your initial photographs, revisit your journal entries, and even consider keeping a checklist of the specific benefits you aimed to achieve. This comprehensive approach will help you see how far you've come and can illuminate the areas where you might wish to focus more attention moving forward.

Finally, remember that tracking progress is not merely about monitoring physical changes but also nurturing a deeper connection with yourself and your body. Embrace the journey, celebrate the small victories, and be kind to yourself throughout the process. Each step you take toward a more natural and holistic approach to health with castor oil will contribute to your overall wellness, cultivating a sense of empowerment and self-awareness.

As you continue to explore the myriad uses of castor oil, allow yourself the grace to adjust your approach and experiment with different remedies. The beauty of this journey lies in its adaptability and the opportunity to learn what resonates most with your unique needs. By diligently tracking your progress and being open to adjusting your routine, you can maximize the benefits of castor oil in your life, paving the way toward a healthier, more vibrant you.

Chapter 11: Holistic Healing: Beyond Castor Oil

Herbalism, often regarded as the oldest form of medicine, is a holistic approach to health and wellness that harnesses the power of nature. It is a practice rooted in traditions that span thousands of years, drawing from the wisdom of various cultures around the globe. While modern medicine has made significant strides, the resurgence of interest in herbal remedies speaks to our innate desire to connect with natural solutions for health concerns. This section will explore the principles of herbalism, its historical significance, and how you can incorporate herbal practices into your everyday life alongside the benefits of castor oil.

At its core, herbalism is the study and use of plants for medicinal purposes. It encompasses a wide range of practices, from the simple use of herbal teas to complex tinctures and extracts. Herbs are recognized not only for their physical healing properties but also for their ability to promote emotional and spiritual well-being. This multifaceted nature of herbalism aligns beautifully with the philosophy of holistic health, which emphasizes the interconnectedness of the body, mind, and spirit.

The history of herbalism is rich and diverse. Ancient civilizations, including the Egyptians, Chinese, Greeks, and Native Americans, relied heavily on plants for healing. The Ebers Papyrus, an Egyptian medical text dating back to around 1550 BC, details over 700 remedies, many of which are based on herbal ingredients. Similarly, Traditional Chinese Medicine (TCM) has a long-standing tradition of using herbs to restore balance and harmony within the body. TCM principles emphasize the importance of understanding the body's energy, or "Qi," and how herbs can play a role in enhancing this vital force.

One of the key aspects of herbalism is the understanding of the individual. Unlike a one-size-fits-all approach often found in conventional medicine, herbalism recognizes that each person is unique, with distinct needs and responses to treatments. This personalized approach is crucial in addressing health concerns comprehensively. Practitioners of herbalism often conduct thorough assessments before recommending specific herbs, taking into account factors such as a person's constitution, lifestyle, and emotional state.

As you embark on your journey with herbalism, you may find it beneficial to familiarize yourself with some of the most common herbs and their uses. For instance, chamomile is widely recognized for its calming effects and is often used to alleviate anxiety and promote restful sleep. Lavender, with its soothing aroma, is not only a popular fragrance but also a potent herb for stress relief and skin health. Echinacea is a well-known immune booster, often employed to fend off colds and infections. Each herb carries its own unique profile of benefits, and learning about them can empower you to make informed choices about your health.

Herbalism also encourages a deep connection with nature. The act of foraging for wild herbs, cultivating a home garden, or simply taking a walk in nature can enhance your understanding of the plants around you. Many herbs can be easily grown in your backyard or even in pots on your windowsill. This connection to the earth deepens your appreciation for the healing properties of plants and allows you to engage actively with your health.

Incorporating herbal remedies alongside your use of castor oil further amplifies your wellness journey. Castor oil itself has a rich history in herbal practices, often regarded as a powerful therapeutic agent. It is not just a standalone remedy; when combined with other herbs, its effects can be enhanced. For example, mixing castor oil with essential oils derived from herbs like rosemary or peppermint can create a potent blend for hair health. Similarly, using castor oil in conjunction with herbal-infused oils, such as calendula or arnica, can offer relief for sore muscles and inflammation.

As you explore the world of herbalism, consider starting a small herbal apothecary at home. This doesn't need to be an elaborate setup; a few well-chosen herbs can serve as the foundation for your natural health toolkit. You might begin with dried herbs, tinctures, or essential oils that resonate with your needs. Over time, you can expand your collection, experimenting with making your own herbal teas, salves, or infused oils.

It's essential to approach herbalism with respect and knowledge. Not all plants are safe for consumption or topical use, and some may interact with medications. It's wise to educate yourself about the herbs you choose to work with, consulting reputable resources or practitioners when needed. Joining local herbalism workshops or online communities can also provide valuable insights and support as you navigate this vast field.

Another vital aspect of herbalism is the emphasis on self-care and mindfulness. The process of preparing herbal remedies can be meditative, allowing you to slow down and connect with your intentions for healing. Whether you are brewing a cup of herbal tea, crafting a healing balm, or simply inhaling the aroma of fresh herbs, these moments can serve as a reminder to honor your body and its needs. This practice of mindfulness complements the use of castor oil, as both approaches encourage a deeper awareness of your health.

As you delve deeper into herbalism, you may find that it opens doors to a broader understanding of health and healing. The principles of herbalism encourage a holistic view, where physical, emotional, and spiritual aspects are intertwined. This perspective aligns seamlessly with the philosophy behind castor oil, as both approaches seek to restore balance and promote wellness naturally.

In conclusion, herbalism is a timeless practice that complements the use of castor oil, offering a path toward a more natural, integrated approach to health. By embracing the wisdom of herbs and understanding their potential, you can empower yourself to take charge of your well-being. Whether you are seeking to address specific health concerns or simply looking to enhance your overall wellness, the world of herbalism holds a treasure trove of knowledge and resources that can enrich your journey. So, as you continue on your path to a healthier, more radiant you, consider the profound connection between nature, herbalism, and the incredible benefits of castor oil.

In our fast-paced, modern world, it's easy to overlook the wisdom that has been passed down through generations, especially when it comes to health and wellness. The ancient practices of holistic healing emphasize the interconnectedness of mind, body, and spirit, offering a comprehensive approach to well-being that transcends isolated treatments. As we delve into natural healing wisdom and practices, it becomes evident that true health is not merely the absence of disease, but a vibrant state of balance.

At the heart of holistic healing is the understanding that our bodies are equipped with innate mechanisms for healing. This self-healing capacity is often hindered by environmental stressors, poor nutrition, and emotional turmoil. By nurturing our bodies through natural remedies, we can tap into this powerful ability. Castor oil, with its multifaceted benefits, serves as an excellent starting point, but it is only one piece of a larger puzzle. Integrating other natural healing practices can enhance its effects and promote a more holistic lifestyle.

One of the cornerstones of natural healing is nutrition. The foods we consume directly impact our health, providing the building blocks for our bodies to function optimally. A diet rich in whole, unprocessed foods—fruits, vegetables, whole grains, nuts, and seeds—can significantly improve our well-being. These foods are packed with essential vitamins, minerals, and antioxidants that help combat inflammation, support digestion, and bolster our immune system. Emphasizing seasonal and locally sourced produce not only nourishes the body but also connects us to our environment, fostering a sense of community and sustainability.

Herbs and spices, much like castor oil, have been used for centuries to support various health concerns. Incorporating herbs such as turmeric, ginger, garlic, and peppermint into your daily routine can provide therapeutic benefits. Turmeric, known for its potent anti-inflammatory properties, can enhance the effects of castor oil when used in conjunction with it, particularly for joint pain or skin conditions. Similarly, ginger aids digestion and can be consumed as a tea or added to meals for an extra health boost. Learning to use these natural ingredients in your cooking not only enhances flavor but also contributes to a more balanced diet.

Movement is another vital component of holistic healing. Engaging in physical activity—whether through yoga, tai chi, dance, or any form of exercise—helps to release tension, improve circulation, and promote mental clarity. The ancient practice of yoga, in particular, emphasizes the connection between breath, body, and mind. By incorporating yoga into your routine, you can cultivate mindfulness and reduce stress, fostering an environment where healing can occur more readily. Additionally, practices such as meditation and deep breathing exercises can help manage stress levels, allowing for a more peaceful state of mind.

Another powerful approach to holistic healing is the concept of energy work. Many traditions recognize the flow of energy within the body, believing that blockages can lead to physical and emotional ailments. Techniques such as acupuncture, Reiki, or even simple practices like visualization can help release these blockages, restoring balance and enhancing overall well-being. By exploring energy work, you may uncover deeper insights into your health and gain tools to empower your healing journey.

Moreover, the power of community and social connections cannot be underestimated in the realm of holistic health. Engaging with supportive networks can provide emotional nourishment, reduce feelings of isolation, and foster a sense of belonging. Whether it's through joining a local wellness group, participating in community events, or simply spending time with loved ones, nurturing relationships can significantly impact your overall health. Sharing experiences, knowledge, and encouragement can create a ripple effect, inspiring others to pursue their own wellness journeys.

As you explore these natural healing practices, it's essential to listen to your body and honor its unique needs. Every individual is different, and what works for one person may not be effective for another. Keeping a wellness journal can be a valuable tool in this regard, allowing you to track your experiences, feelings, and progress. Documenting how various practices affect your well-being can help you identify what resonates most with you, guiding you toward a personalized holistic healing path.

Integrating castor oil into your daily routine can serve as a catalyst for embracing these natural healing wisdoms. For example, using castor oil in a massage can enhance the benefits of physical touch, promoting relaxation and reducing muscle tension. Pairing castor oil with herbal infusions can create potent topical remedies that address specific skin concerns, while also encouraging a mindful self-care ritual.

Ultimately, the journey of holistic healing is a lifelong process that encourages exploration, experimentation, and self-discovery. By embracing the wisdom of natural remedies and practices, you empower yourself to take charge of your health and well-being. The beauty of this journey lies in its flexibility; you can adapt and evolve your practices as you learn and grow.

In this quest for holistic health, remember to approach every aspect of your life with intention. Whether it's the food you eat, the movement you practice, or the thoughts you cultivate, each choice plays a role in shaping your overall well-being. By weaving together the threads of nutrition, movement, energy work, and community, you create a rich tapestry of health that not only nourishes your body but also uplifts your spirit.

As you continue to explore the benefits of castor oil alongside these holistic practices, you'll find that your journey toward wellness becomes not just a series of isolated actions, but a harmonious way of living that celebrates the intricate connections between all aspects of your life. Embrace this journey with an open heart and mind, and allow the natural healing wisdom to guide you toward a healthier, more vibrant you.

In the quest for holistic healing, it's essential to recognize that no single remedy holds all the answers. Nature has bestowed upon us a treasure trove of plants, herbs, and oils, each with unique properties that can address various health concerns. Integrating multiple remedies into your wellness routine can create a synergistic effect, enhancing your overall health and well-being. This approach not only diversifies your treatment options but also allows you to tailor your healing journey to your individual needs.

When we think of holistic healing, we often envision a harmonious balance between the mind, body, and spirit. This balance is best achieved by combining different natural remedies, each supporting the other in a beautiful tapestry of health. For instance, while castor oil is a powerful ally for skin rejuvenation and pain relief, it can be even more effective when paired with complementary ingredients, such as essential oils or herbal infusions.

One effective way to integrate multiple remedies is through the art of blending. For skin care, consider mixing castor oil with tea tree oil, known for its antibacterial properties. This combination can help treat acne-prone skin, as castor oil hydrates and nourishes while tea tree oil combats breakouts. Similarly, adding a few drops of lavender essential oil can provide additional soothing benefits, promoting relaxation and reducing inflammation.

In your hair care routine, castor oil can be mixed with coconut oil, another natural powerhouse known for its deep conditioning capabilities. Together, they can create a nourishing hair mask that stimulates growth, reduces protein loss, and restores shine. Adding a few drops of rosemary essential oil can further enhance this mixture, as it is believed to stimulate hair follicles and improve circulation to the scalp.

Beyond topical applications, the integration of remedies extends to dietary choices and holistic practices. If you're focusing on gut health, for example, consider complementing castor oil's detoxifying effects with foods rich in probiotics, such as yogurt or fermented vegetables. This combination can help restore balance in your digestive system, promoting a healthy gut flora that aids in nutrient absorption and overall wellness.

Herbal teas can also play a significant role in your holistic healing regimen. Chamomile tea can be a calming addition when used alongside castor oil for alleviating menstrual cramps. The anti-inflammatory properties of chamomile combined with the soothing effects of castor oil create a powerful duo for managing discomfort. Similarly, ginger tea, known for its ability to alleviate nausea and support digestion, can complement the detoxifying properties of castor oil, enhancing your body's natural cleansing processes.

When integrating multiple remedies, it's crucial to be mindful of the timing and method of administration. For instance, if you're taking castor oil orally for digestive issues, consider the timing of your meals. It's best to take it on an empty stomach or at least an hour before or after eating to maximize its effects. Pairing it with herbal teas or warming spices, such as cinnamon or turmeric, can enhance its digestive benefits and make the experience more enjoyable.

Another important aspect of integrating remedies involves understanding the principles of synergy. Certain combinations can amplify each other's effects, leading to more significant results than when used in isolation. For example, combining castor oil with honey not only increases the moisture content of your skin but also provides antibacterial properties, making it an excellent option for treating wounds and blemishes. The natural humectant properties of honey work in tandem with castor oil's nourishing qualities, creating a dynamic duo for skin health.

Incorporating lifestyle changes can also enhance the benefits of these natural remedies. Regular exercise, mindfulness practices, and a balanced diet can all support your body's healing process. For instance, yoga or gentle stretches can complement the pain relief benefits of castor oil by promoting flexibility and circulation. Pairing physical activity with a restorative approach to self-care, such as using castor oil packs to ease muscle tension, can yield remarkable results.

Listening to your body is vital in this integrative approach. Everyone's body responds differently to various remedies, so it's essential to pay attention to how you feel after incorporating new elements into your routine. Keeping a journal to track your experiences can be beneficial. Note any changes in symptoms, energy levels, or overall well-being. This practice not only helps you identify what works best for you but also empowers you to take charge of your health journey.

As you explore the world of holistic healing, remember that patience is key. Natural remedies often require time to work their magic, and results may not be immediate. Celebrate small victories along the way, whether it's improved skin clarity, increased energy, or reduced discomfort. Each step forward is a testament to your commitment to nurturing your health naturally.

Lastly, consider the power of community in your holistic healing journey. Sharing experiences and advice with others who are also exploring natural remedies can provide valuable insights and encouragement. Online forums, local workshops, or even social media groups can connect you with like-minded individuals eager to share their successes and challenges. This sense of community can foster accountability and motivation, making your journey toward holistic well-being more enriching.

By integrating multiple remedies into your daily routine, you can create a personalized approach to health that resonates with your unique needs. Castor oil serves as a brilliant foundation, but the possibilities are endless when you combine it with other natural remedies. Embrace the synergy of nature's offerings, nurture your body's innate healing abilities, and embark on a transformative path toward lasting wellness. Remember, holistic healing is not just about addressing symptoms; it's about cultivating a deeper connection with yourself and the world around you, allowing for a more vibrant and fulfilling life.

Chapter 12: Real-Life Transformations

The journey to embracing natural remedies can often feel daunting, especially when so many products on the market promise results but fail to deliver. However, the success stories of individuals who have integrated castor oil into their routines can serve as powerful motivators. These testimonies not only highlight the versatility of castor oil but also illustrate its profound impact on a wide range of health and beauty concerns.

Take the story of Sarah, a 34-year-old graphic designer from Austin, Texas. For years, Sarah struggled with acne and the scars that accompanied it. She had tried countless treatments, from prescription creams to expensive facials, but nothing seemed to work. After discovering "The Castor Oil Bible," Sarah was intrigued by the section on DIY treatments for acne. With a mix of skepticism and hope, she decided to give it a try.

Following the recipes in the book, Sarah created a simple yet effective face mask using castor oil combined with honey and lemon juice. She applied it twice a week, and within a month, she noticed a significant reduction in her breakouts. Not only did her skin clear up, but the scars began to fade as well. "I couldn't believe how something so simple could change my skin," she shared. "It's like I finally found the missing piece to my skincare routine."

Then there's James, a 45-year-old father of two, who had been battling thinning hair for the better part of a decade. He felt self-conscious and frustrated, often opting for hats to hide his receding hairline. When he stumbled upon the chapter dedicated to transforming hair with castor oil, he felt a flicker of hope. The idea of stimulating hair growth naturally appealed to him, especially since he wanted to avoid harsh chemicals.

James diligently followed the advice in the book, incorporating castor oil into his nightly routine by massaging it into his scalp. He also experimented with the homemade hair masks suggested in the recipes section, combining castor oil with coconut oil and essential oils for added nourishment. After several weeks, he began to notice tiny new hairs sprouting along his hairline. "It was a gradual process, but seeing those little hairs was like a light at the end of the tunnel," James recounted. "Now, I feel more confident and even started experimenting with different hairstyles."

Transformations aren't limited to skin and hair; they can also encompass overall wellness. Maria, a 29-year-old yoga instructor, had long struggled with digestive issues that left her feeling bloated and uncomfortable. After reading about the detox benefits of castor oil, she decided to incorporate it into her routine. Following the guidance in the book, she started with a teaspoon of castor oil mixed with warm water on an empty stomach each morning.

Within a few days, Maria experienced a noticeable improvement in her digestion. "I can't even describe how liberating it felt to finally have a solution to my bloating," she said with a smile. "I was able to focus on my yoga practice without discomfort, and my energy levels skyrocketed." Her experience inspired her to share her newfound wisdom with her yoga community, encouraging others to explore natural remedies.

Another remarkable story comes from Linda, a 52-year-old woman who had been grappling with chronic joint pain for years. Having tried various over-the-counter medications with limited results, she was hesitant about using castor oil for pain relief. However, after reading testimonials in “The Castor Oil Bible,” she decided to give it a shot.

Linda followed the section on pain and inflammation relief, applying a castor oil compress to her knees every evening. To her amazement, she found that her discomfort began to diminish within a matter of days. “I felt like I was finally reclaiming my life,” Linda recalled. “I could play with my grandchildren again without wincing in pain. It was a game-changer for me.” She now swears by castor oil and has even inspired others in her book club to explore its benefits.

The impact of castor oil extends beyond individual transformations; it fosters a sense of community among those who seek natural solutions. In a small town in Oregon, a group of friends formed a “Castor Oil Club” after discovering the book together. They began meeting weekly to share recipes and experiences, each woman bringing her unique insights into how castor oil had benefited her life. From skincare to hair care and even crafting, their discussions turned into a celebration of holistic wellness.

These testimonials illustrate that the journey to health and beauty through natural remedies is not just about the results; it’s about the empowerment that comes with discovering effective solutions. The stories of Sarah, James, Maria, and Linda remind us that castor oil is more than just an ingredient; it’s a bridge to reclaiming self-confidence and well-being.

As you consider your own journey with castor oil, remember that these transformations are achievable. The experiences shared by others serve as a testament to the potential that lies within this golden oil and the power of embracing natural remedies. By integrating castor oil into your daily routine, you too can discover the profound impact it can have on your skin, hair, health, and overall sense of self. The journey may be unique to you, but the potential for transformation is limitless.

The power of transformation is not just a concept; it's a reality vividly illustrated through the inspiring stories of individuals who have embraced the wonders of castor oil. These transformations are captured not only in words but also through compelling visuals that showcase the dramatic changes in skin, hair, and overall wellness. Before and after images serve as a testament to the efficacy of this natural remedy, revealing the profound impact it can have when integrated into daily routines.

Take, for instance, the story of Emily, a 32-year-old woman who struggled with chronic acne for most of her adult life. Years of battling blemishes led her to try a myriad of treatments, from harsh chemical peels to expensive dermatological procedures. Frustrated by the lack of lasting results and the side effects of many products, Emily turned to castor oil after reading about its myriad benefits. In her before photo, her skin was marked by redness and inflammation, common side effects of the treatments she had endured. However, after just eight weeks of using a simple nightly castor oil regimen, Emily's transformation was remarkable. Her after photo radiated a glow she had long thought impossible, with minimized scars and a clear complexion. Emily described her journey as liberating—not only did she find a solution that worked, but she also gained confidence in her natural beauty.

Then there's Michael, who faced thinning hair and a receding hairline at an early age. He had tried numerous shampoos and topical treatments with little success, often feeling defeated by societal standards of masculinity tied to a full head of hair. When he discovered the hair growth properties of castor oil, he decided to give it a chance. In his before image, the top of his head looked sparse and lifeless. A few months into his castor oil treatment, Michael documented his progress, showcasing his fuller hair and healthier scalp. His after image, brimming with vitality, captures his newfound pride in his appearance. Michael shared how this transformation not only rejuvenated his hair but also restored his self-esteem, empowering him to embrace his individuality.

The power of castor oil extends beyond beauty; it touches the lives of those seeking relief from chronic pain. Sarah, a 45-year-old yoga instructor, had long been plagued by joint pain that limited her mobility and enthusiasm for her passion. She had turned to over-the-counter pain relievers and topical creams, all of which offered temporary relief at best. After integrating castor oil into her wellness routine—specifically as a soothing massage oil—she experienced gradual improvement. Her before photo captured a moment of discomfort, her face reflecting the strain of living with persistent pain. In her stunning after image, however, there's a palpable sense of joy and freedom as she effortlessly moves through a yoga pose, showcasing not just a physical transformation but a holistic revival of her spirit.

Real-life transformations also highlight the emotional and psychological impact of embracing natural remedies. Lisa, who faced emotional distress due to her struggle with cellulite and stretch marks, found solace in castor oil. The before image depicts her visible unease, a snapshot of self-doubt and frustration. After incorporating castor oil into her body care routine, the after photo reveals a confident Lisa, unafraid to flaunt her skin. Her radiant smile tells a story of acceptance and love for her body, showcasing how addressing physical concerns can lead to profound internal changes.

As you look at these visual transformations, it’s essential to acknowledge that each journey is unique. The stories of Emily, Michael, Sarah, and Lisa illustrate a common thread: the transition from frustration to empowerment through the natural healing properties of castor oil. They remind us that beauty and wellness should not come at the expense of our health or self-esteem. Instead, they inspire a movement towards embracing what nature offers in a world often dominated by synthetic solutions.

These transformations also bring forth a broader community of individuals who have come together to share their experiences, providing support and encouragement. The before and after visuals they share are more than mere photographs; they symbolize hope, resilience, and the triumph of natural healing. Through social media platforms and community forums, testimonials and images have helped cultivate a supportive environment where individuals can exchange tips, recipes, and results, creating a sense of belonging among those on similar journeys.

As you embark on your own path with castor oil, remember that change takes time. The journey may have its ups and downs, but the stories of transformation remind us that perseverance pays off. The before and after visuals are not just milestones; they are celebrations of personal growth, a testament that embracing natural remedies can lead to lasting change in both our appearance and our well-being.

Incorporating castor oil isn’t merely about following a trend; it's about forging a connection with nature's gifts and rediscovering our innate ability to heal and rejuvenate. As you flip through the pages of this book and explore the recipes and insights provided, envision the before and after visuals that will tell your story. Picture the radiance of your skin, the vitality of your hair, and the ease of movement that comes with relief from discomfort. With each application, you're not just applying oil; you're participating in a transformative journey toward a healthier, more vibrant you.

In our journey towards embracing the natural wonders of castor oil, one of the most empowering aspects lies in the sense of community and ongoing support that can significantly enhance our experiences. When we embark on a new path—especially one that involves making changes to our health and beauty routines—it can be incredibly beneficial to surround ourselves with others who are on a similar journey. This shared experience not only fosters motivation but also provides a wealth of knowledge, encouragement, and inspiration.

As you begin to incorporate castor oil into your daily life, consider seeking out groups or forums that focus on natural remedies and holistic wellness. Online platforms, social media groups, and local community workshops are excellent resources for connecting with like-minded individuals who share your interests. These communities often serve as a safe space for sharing experiences, asking questions, and exchanging tips and tricks. Whether you're looking for advice on specific castor oil applications or seeking reassurance during your journey, knowing that you are not alone can be immensely comforting.

Engaging with a supportive community allows you to witness the transformations of others, fueling your own motivation. When you see real-life examples of people who have experienced positive changes—whether it's glowing skin, healthier hair, or relief from chronic pain—it reinforces the belief that these benefits are attainable for you as well. Celebrating these successes together creates a bond that can uplift everyone involved.

Moreover, sharing your own experiences can be just as rewarding. As you start to notice changes in your own body, whether it's a reduction in acne or an increase in hair thickness, documenting your journey not only helps you track your progress but also encourages others who may be struggling. Your story could inspire someone else to take the leap toward natural wellness. In this way, community support becomes a cycle of encouragement, where sharing personal victories and challenges fosters an atmosphere of growth and healing.

To enhance your experience with castor oil, consider starting a journal. This can be a private space or one shared with your community. In it, you can document your discoveries, recipes that worked for you, and even setbacks. By reflecting on your journey, you create a roadmap that can guide you through the ups and downs of transitioning to natural remedies. Sharing snippets of your journal with your community can spark conversations and lead to valuable exchanges of information.

Additionally, consider participating in local workshops or classes that focus on natural remedies. Many communities offer sessions on herbalism, DIY beauty products, and holistic health practices, all of which can complement your castor oil regimen. These in-person events provide an opportunity to connect with others face-to-face, ask questions, and learn hands-on techniques that enhance your understanding of natural health.

Social media platforms are another effective way to cultivate ongoing support. Instagram, Facebook, and Pinterest are filled with influencers and enthusiasts who share their experiences with castor oil and other natural remedies. Following these accounts allows you to stay updated on the latest trends, tips, and scientific findings related to herbs and oils. You can also participate in challenges, such as a "30-day castor oil challenge," where participants commit to using castor oil daily and share their results. Such initiatives not only keep you accountable but also enrich your journey through collective motivation.

For those who prefer more structured support, consider joining online courses or webinars that delve deeper into the properties and applications of castor oil. Many experts offer courses that cover a range of topics, from skincare to pain relief, specifically focusing on natural remedies. Engaging in these educational experiences not only expands your knowledge but also connects you with fellow learners who share your passion for natural health.

It's also essential to remember that support doesn't always have to come from a community of individuals. You might find mentors or health practitioners who specialize in natural remedies and holistic health. Their guidance can provide you with customized advice based on your unique needs, helping you navigate any challenges you may encounter. These professionals can serve as valuable resources for troubleshooting any issues and offer insights that may not be readily available in community forums.

As you progress in your journey with castor oil, consider giving back to the community that has supported you. Sharing your knowledge, experiences, and even your homemade recipes can empower others who are just starting out. Whether it's through social media posts, blog entries, or local meetups, your contributions can inspire others to explore the transformative power of castor oil.

Moreover, organizing or participating in local meetups dedicated to natural health can foster a sense of camaraderie among participants. Such gatherings allow for the exchange of ideas, recipes, and personal stories, creating a rich tapestry of collective knowledge and support. You can even host workshops to teach others how to use castor oil effectively, further solidifying your role as a community leader and advocate for natural remedies.

Ultimately, the journey with castor oil is not just about personal transformation; it is about building connections and fostering a supportive environment that encourages exploration and discovery. By engaging with community, sharing victories and setbacks, and offering support to others, you create an enriching and empowering experience that enhances not only your wellness journey but also the journeys of those around you.

Remember, healing is not a solitary path. Together, we can celebrate our successes, learn from our challenges, and empower each other to embrace the natural remedies that can lead us to healthier, more vibrant lives. As you continue to explore the myriad ways castor oil can benefit you, keep in mind that the connections you forge are just as vital as the remedies themselves. Embrace the journey, lean on your community, and watch as the transformative power of castor oil unfolds in your life.

www.ingramcontent.com/pod-product-compliance
Lightning Source LLC
LaVergne TN
LVHW022102200926
848481LV00003B/1038

* 9 7 9 8 8 9 8 4 3 1 5 8 7 *